Welcome to ***"110+ Recipes Cookbook for Young Chefs: Simple Step-by-Step Instructions for Aspiring Cooks"!***

This cookbook is designed to inspire and guide young chefs on a culinary adventure, providing a wide range of delicious and easy-to-make recipes that will help you develop your cooking skills and confidence in the kitchen. Whether you're a beginner just starting out or have some experience and are looking to expand your repertoire, this book has something for everyone.

Why Cooking?

Cooking is not just about preparing food—it's an essential life skill that can bring joy, creativity, and independence. As you learn to cook, you'll discover the pleasure of creating something delicious from scratch, the satisfaction of sharing a meal with family and friends, and the pride that comes with mastering new techniques and recipes.

What to Expect

In this cookbook, you'll find over 110 recipes, carefully selected to suit young chefs. Each recipe includes simple, step-by-step instructions, clear ingredient lists, and helpful tips to ensure your success. From breakfast to dinner, snacks to desserts, there's a wide variety of dishes to explore, each designed to be fun and accessible.

Highlights of the Book

- Easy and Fun Meals: Recipes that are straightforward and enjoyable to make.

- Healthy Choices: Nutritious options to help you build a balanced diet.

- Creative Recipes: Dishes that encourage you to experiment with new flavors and techniques.

- Family-Friendly:Meals that are perfect for cooking and sharing with your loved ones.

- Step-by-Step Guidance: Detailed instructions to help you every step of the way.

Getting Started

Before you dive into the recipes, take some time to familiarize yourself with the basics of kitchen safety, essential cooking tools, and common ingredients. We've included a section at the beginning of the book to help you get started on the right foot.

Thank you for choosing this cookbook as your guide. We hope it brings you as much joy in cooking as we've had in creating it for you. Now, let's get cooking and start making delicious memories!

1. SCRAMBLED EGGS

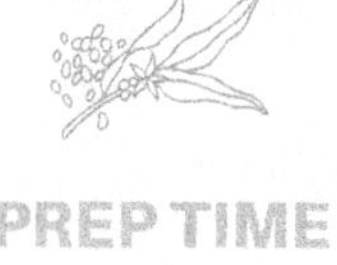

PREP TIME
20 MINUTES

COOK TIME
30 MINUTES

INGREDIENTS:

• 2 eggs
• 1 tbsp milk or water
• 1/2 tsp butter or oil
• Pinch of salt and pepper
(optional)

PROCEDURE:

1. Crack the 2 eggs into a small bowl. Add the milk or water and a pinch of salt and pepper if desired. Use a fork to beat the eggs until well mixed.

2. Heat a small non•stick skillet over medium heat and add the butter or oil.

3. When the pan is hot, pour in the beaten eggs. Use a spatula to gently push and fold the eggs as they cook, creating soft, fluffy curds.

4. Cook the eggs, folding and stirring occasionally, until they are softly set, about 2•3 minutes total.

5. Remove the pan from the heat and serve the scrambled eggs immediately.

Tips for young chefs:
• Crack the eggs carefully to avoid getting any shell in the bowl.
• Use a fork or whisk to beat the eggs until they are well blended.
• Move the spatula slowly and gently to avoid over•stirring the eggs.
• Watch the eggs closely as they cook to prevent them from overcooking.

Enjoy your delicious homemade scrambled eggs!

2. PANCAKES

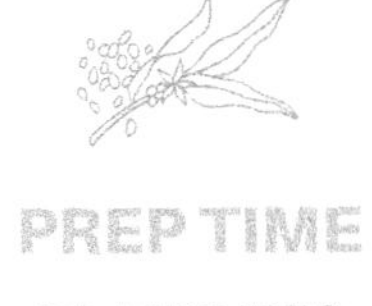

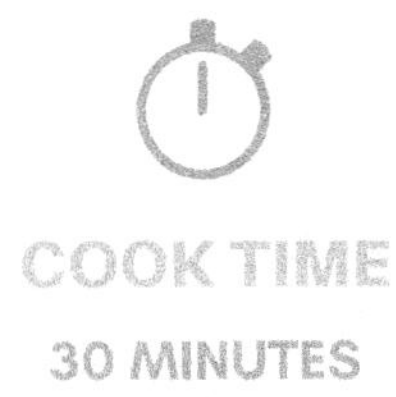

PREP TIME
20 MINUTES

COOK TIME
30 MINUTES

INGREDIENTS:

• 1 cup all•purpose flour
• 2 teaspoons baking powder
• 1 tablespoon sugar
• 1/4 teaspoon salt
• 1 egg
• 1 cup milk
• 2 tablespoons melted butter or oil

Tips for young chefs:
• Measure the ingredients carefully for best results.
• Avoid overmixing the batter, which can make the pancakes tough.
• Use a ladle or measuring cup to portion out the batter onto the griddle.
• Watch the pancakes closely as they cook to prevent burning.
• Get an adult to help with the hot griddle or skillet.

PROCEDURE:

1. In a medium bowl, whisk together the flour, baking powder, sugar, and salt.

2. In a separate bowl, beat the egg. Then stir in the milk and melted butter or oil.

3. Pour the wet ingredients into the dry ingredients and stir just until combined (do not overmix).

4. Heat a lightly oiled griddle or non•stick skillet over medium heat.

5. For each pancake, pour about 1/4 cup of batter onto the griddle. Cook until bubbles appear on the surface, about 2•3 minutes.

6. Flip the pancake and cook until golden brown on the other side, about 1•2 minutes more.

7. Serve the pancakes warm, with your favorite toppings like syrup, fruit, whipped cream, etc.

Enjoy your homemade pancakes!

3. FRENCH TOAST

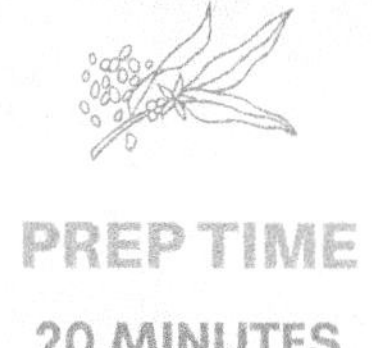 

PREP TIME
20 MINUTES

COOK TIME
30 MINUTES

INGREDIENTS:

• 3 eggs
• 1/2 cup milk
• 1 teaspoon vanilla extract
• 1/4 teaspoon ground cinnamon (optional)
• 4•6 slices of bread
• Butter or oil for cooking

Tips for young chefs:

• Use day•old or slightly stale bread for best results.
• Dip the bread slices in the egg mixture just before cooking to prevent them from getting soggy.
• Adjust the heat as needed to prevent the French toast from burning.
• Be careful when flipping the slices to avoid breaking them.
• Get an adult to help with the hot cooking surface.

PROCEDURE:

1. In a shallow bowl, whisk together the eggs, milk, vanilla, and cinnamon (if using).

2. Dip each slice of bread into the egg mixture, coating both sides evenly.

3. Heat a skillet or griddle over medium heat and add a small amount of butter or oil.

4. Place the soaked bread slices onto the hot surface and cook for 2•3 minutes per side, until golden brown.

5. Flip the slices carefully using a spatula. Cook the other side until it's also golden brown.

6. Serve the French toast warm, with your favorite toppings like syrup, powdered sugar, fruit, or whipped cream.

Enjoy your homemade French toast!

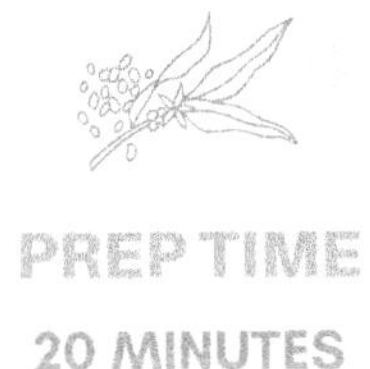

4. SMOOTHIE BOWLS

PREP TIME
20 MINUTES

COOK TIME
30 MINUTES

INGREDIENTS:

- 1 cup frozen fruit (such as berries, banana, mango)
- 1/2 cup milk or non•dairy milk
- 1/4 cup yogurt (optional)
- 1 tablespoon honey or maple syrup (optional)
- Toppings (such as fresh fruit, granola, nuts, seeds)

PROCEDURE:

1. In a blender, combine the frozen fruit, milk, yogurt (if using), and honey or maple syrup (if using). Blend until smooth and creamy.

2. Pour the smoothie into a bowl.

3. Top the smoothie with your favorite toppings, such as:
- Fresh fruit (sliced banana, berries, kiwi, etc.)
- Granola or crunchy cereal
- Nuts or seeds (sliced almonds, chia seeds, etc.)
- A drizzle of honey or nut butter

Tips for young chefs:
- Use frozen fruit for a thick, creamy smoothie. You can use fresh fruit too, but you may need to add ice cubes.
- Start with a small amount of liquid and add more as needed to get the desired consistency.
- Let the blender run for a minute or two to ensure the smoothie is well blended.
- Get creative with the toppings! Try different fruits, nuts, seeds, and other fun additions.
- Ask an adult for help when using the blender, as the blades can be sharp.

Enjoy your colorful and nutritious smoothie bowl!

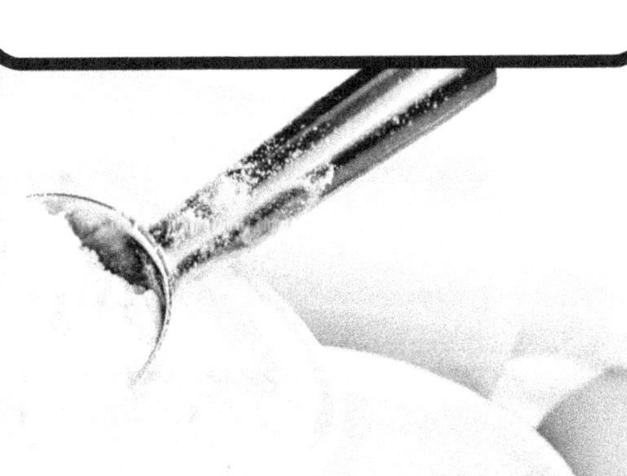

5. OMELETS

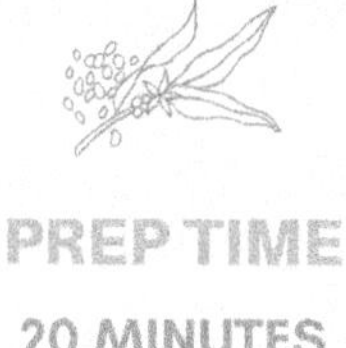 

PREP TIME
20 MINUTES

COOK TIME
30 MINUTES

INGREDIENTS:

- 2 eggs
- 1 tablespoon milk or water
- 1/2 tablespoon butter or oil
- Salt and pepper to taste
- Optional fillings: cheese, diced vegetables, cooked meat, etc.

Tips for young chefs:

- Crack the eggs carefully to avoid getting any shell in the bowl.
- Use a fork or whisk to beat the eggs until they are well blended.
- Move the spatula slowly and gently to avoid over•stirring the eggs.
- Watch the eggs closely as they cook to prevent them from overcooking.
- Be creative with the fillings • try cheese, veggies, ham, etc.
- Get an adult to help with the hot pan.

PROCEDURE:

1. Crack the 2 eggs into a small bowl. Add the milk or water and a pinch of salt and pepper. Use a fork to beat the eggs until well mixed.

2. Heat a small non•stick skillet over medium heat and add the butter or oil.

3. When the pan is hot, pour in the beaten eggs. Use a spatula to gently push and fold the eggs as they cook, creating soft, fluffy curds.

4. When the eggs are mostly set but still a bit wet on top, add your desired fillings to one half of the omelet.

5. Use the spatula to fold the unfilled half of the omelet over the filled half.

6. Cook for another 30 seconds to 1 minute, then slide the omelet onto a plate.

Enjoy your delicious homemade omelet!

6. BREAKFAST BURRITOS

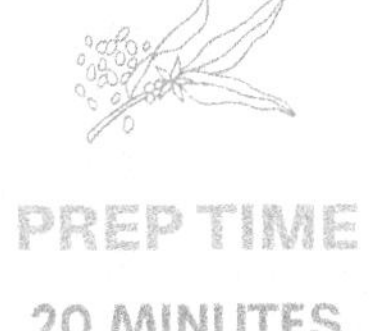 

PREP TIME
20 MINUTES

COOK TIME
30 MINUTES

INGREDIENTS:

- 4 eggs
- 2 tablespoons milk
- 1 tablespoon butter or oil
- 1/4 cup shredded cheese (such as cheddar or pepper jack)
- 4 small flour tortillas
- Optional fillings: cooked bacon or sausage, diced bell peppers, onions, spinach, etc.

Tips for young chefs:

- Crack the eggs carefully to avoid getting any shell in the bowl.
- Use a spatula to gently stir the eggs as they cook to create soft, fluffy curds.
- Be careful when handling the hot skillet.
- Warm the tortillas so they are pliable and easy to roll.
- Get creative with the fillings • try cooked meats, veggies, or even hash browns!
- Ask an adult for help with any steps that involve heat or sharp tools.

PROCEDURE:

1. In a small bowl, whisk together the eggs and milk. Season with a pinch of salt and pepper.

2. Heat a non•stick skillet over medium heat and melt the butter or oil.

3. Pour the egg mixture into the hot skillet and let it cook, stirring occasionally, until the eggs are softly scrambled, about 2•3 minutes.

4. Remove the scrambled eggs from the heat and stir in the shredded cheese.

5. Warm the tortillas according to package instructions, or briefly in the microwave or a dry skillet.

6. Spoon the cheesy scrambled eggs onto the center of each tortilla. Add any additional fillings you desire.

7. Fold the bottom of the tortilla up, then fold in the sides and continue rolling up tightly to create a burrito.

8. Serve the breakfast burritos warm.

Enjoy your homemade breakfast burritos!

7. GRANOLA AND YOGURT PARFAITS

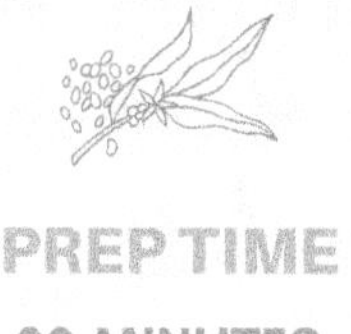

PREP TIME

20 MINUTES

COOK TIME

30 MINUTES

INGREDIENTS :

- 1 cup plain Greek yogurt
- 1/2 cup granola
- 1 cup fresh or frozen berries (such as strawberries, blueberries, raspberries)
- 1•2 teaspoons honey (optional)

PROCEDURE :

1. In a clear glass or jar, layer the ingredients in the following order:
   - 1/4 cup of yogurt
   - 2•3 tablespoons of granola
   - 1/4 cup of berries

2. Repeat the layers, ending with a layer of yogurt on top.

3. If desired, drizzle a small amount of honey over the top of the parfait.

4. Serve immediately or refrigerate until ready to eat.

Tips for young chefs:

- Use your favorite flavors of yogurt and granola.
- Try different types of fresh or frozen berries for variety.
- Adjust the amounts of each ingredient to your taste preferences.
- Get creative with the layering • you can make multiple layers in a tall glass or just a single layer in a bowl.
- Ask an adult for help when using any sharp tools or the refrigerator.
- Enjoy your healthy and delicious parfait!

8. BANANA BREAD

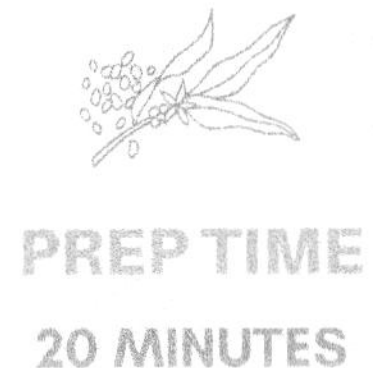

PREP TIME	COOK TIME
20 MINUTES	30 MINUTES

INGREDIENTS:

- 1 1/2 cups all•purpose flour
- 1 teaspoon baking soda
- 1/4 teaspoon salt
- 1/2 cup unsalted butter, softened
- 3/4 cup granulated sugar
- 2 large eggs
- 1 teaspoon vanilla extract
- 1 1/4 cups mashed ripe bananas (about 3 medium bananas)

Tips for young chefs:

- Use very ripe, spotty bananas for the best flavor.
- Mash the bananas well with a fork or potato masher.
- Be careful not to overmix the batter, as this can make the bread tough.
- Use an oven mitt or ask an adult for help when removing the hot loaf pan from the oven.
- Let the bread cool completely before slicing to prevent it from crumbling.
- Enjoy your delicious homemade banana bread!

PROCEDURE:

1. Preheat your oven to 350°F (175°C). Grease a 9x5 inch loaf pan with butter or non•stick cooking spray.

2. In a medium bowl, whisk together the flour, baking soda, and salt. Set aside.

3. In a large bowl, use a hand mixer or a wooden spoon to cream the softened butter and sugar together until light and fluffy, about 2•3 minutes.

4. Beat in the eggs one at a time, then stir in the vanilla extract and mashed bananas until well combined.

5. Gradually add the dry ingredients to the wet ingredients, mixing just until incorporated. Be careful not to overmix.

6. Pour the batter into the prepared loaf pan and smooth the top with a spatula.

7. Bake for 55•65 minutes, or until a toothpick inserted in the center comes out clean.

8. Allow the banana bread to cool in the pan for 10 minutes, then transfer it to a wire rack to cool completely before slicing.

9. AVOCADO TOAST

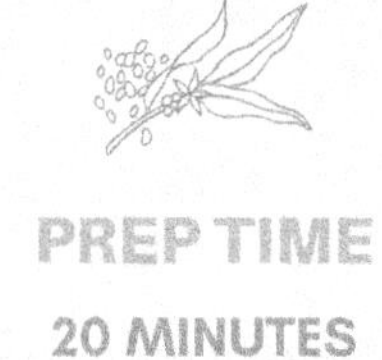 

PREP TIME
20 MINUTES

COOK TIME
30 MINUTES

INGREDIENTS:

- 1 ripe avocado
- 2 slices of whole grain or sourdough bread
- 1 tablespoon olive oil or butter
- Salt and pepper to taste
- Optional toppings: cherry tomatoes, sliced radish, crumbled feta, everything bagel seasoning, etc.

Tips for young chefs:
- Choose a ripe avocado that is soft but not mushy.
- Be careful when cutting the avocado in half and removing the pit.
- Use a fork or the back of a spoon to mash the avocado, leaving it a bit chunky.
- Toast the bread until it's crispy but not burnt.
- Get creative with different topping combinations.
- Ask an adult for help with any sharp tools or hot surfaces.

PROCEDURE:

1. Toast the bread slices until lightly golden brown.

2. While the bread is toasting, cut the avocado in half lengthwise and remove the pit. Scoop the avocado flesh into a small bowl.

3. Use a fork to mash the avocado until it's slightly chunky. You can also use the back of a spoon to mash it.

4. Spread the mashed avocado evenly over the toasted bread slices.

5. Drizzle a small amount of olive oil or dot with a bit of butter over the avocado.

6. Season with a pinch of salt and pepper.

7. If desired, top the avocado toast with any additional toppings like cherry tomatoes, sliced radish, crumbled feta, or a sprinkle of everything bagel seasoning.

Enjoy your delicious and nutritious avocado toast!

10. FRUIT SALAD

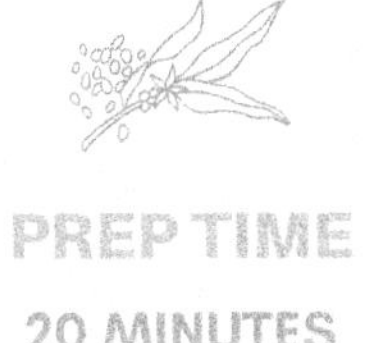

PREP TIME
20 MINUTES

COOK TIME
30 MINUTES

INGREDIENTS:

- 1 cup diced strawberries
- 1 cup diced pineapple
- 1 cup diced mango
- 1 cup diced kiwi
- 1 tablespoon honey (optional)

This refreshing and healthy fruit salad is a great way for young chefs to practice their knife skills and explore new fruits.

PROCEDURE:

1. Wash all the fruit and pat it dry with a paper towel.

2. Use a child•safe knife or plastic knife to carefully cut the fruit into bite•sized pieces.

3. Place the diced fruit in a large bowl and gently mix them together.

4. If desired, drizzle the honey over the fruit salad and stir to coat.

Tips for young chefs:

- Let the kids help wash and cut the fruit. Supervise them when using any sharp knives.
- Encourage them to try different types of fruit, such as grapes, blueberries, or melon.
- Suggest they arrange the fruit in a fun pattern or design in the bowl.
- Discuss the importance of eating a variety of colorful fruits.
- Remind them to wash their hands before and after handling the fruit.
- Offer a small spoon or fork for them to serve the fruit salad.
- Explain that the honey is optional and can be left out if they prefer.

11. PEANUT BUTTER AND JELLY SANDWICHES

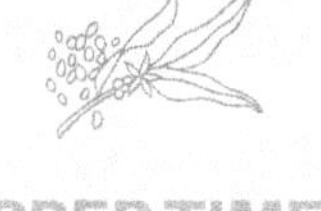 

PREP TIME
20 MINUTES

COOK TIME
30 MINUTES

INGREDIENTS :

- 2 slices of whole wheat or white bread
- 2 tablespoons peanut butter
- 2 tablespoons jelly or jam

Tips for young chefs:

- Let the kids help measure and spread the peanut butter and jelly.

- Encourage them to use different types of bread, such as whole wheat, white, or even bagels.

- Suggest they try different flavors of jelly or jam, like strawberry, grape, or raspberry.

- Remind them to use a clean knife and to spread the ingredients to the edges of the bread.

PROCEDURE :

1. Gather all the ingredients and place them on a clean, flat surface.

2. Using a butter knife, spread the peanut butter evenly on one slice of bread.

3. On the other slice of bread, spread the jelly or jam evenly.

4. Carefully place the peanut butter side and the jelly side together to create a sandwich.

5. Cut the sandwich in half, diagonally or straight across, if desired.

- Discuss the importance of food safety, such as washing hands before handling food.

- Offer other toppings like banana slices, honey, or sprinkles to make the sandwiches more fun.

- Supervise young chefs when using knives or other sharp tools.

This classic sandwich is a great way for young chefs to practice their sandwich•making skills and explore different flavor combinations.

12. HOMEMADE TRAIL MIX

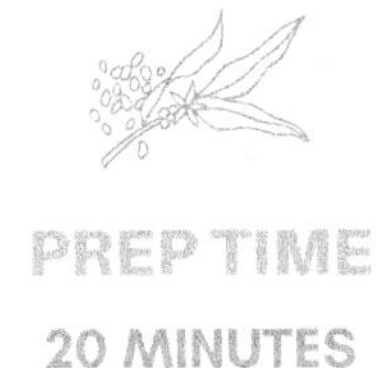

PREP TIME
20 MINUTES

COOK TIME
30 MINUTES

INGREDIENTS :

• 1 cup roasted, unsalted nuts (such as almonds, cashews, or peanuts)
• 1/2 cup dried fruit (such as raisins, cranberries, or apricots)
• 1/2 cup whole grain cereal or granola
• 1/4 cup seeds (such as sunflower or pumpkin seeds)
• 1/4 cup dark chocolate chips or carob chips (optional)

This homemade trail mix is a great way for young chefs to learn about healthy snacking and get creative in the kitchen.

PROCEDURE :

1. In a large bowl, combine all the ingredients and mix well.

2. Divide the trail mix into individual servings in small containers or bags.

Tips for young chefs:

• Let the kids help measure and pour the ingredients into the bowl.

• Encourage them to choose their favorite nuts, dried fruits, and other mix•ins.

• Discuss the importance of a balanced, healthy snack with protein, fiber, and healthy fats.

• Remind them to wash their hands before handling the food.

• Supervise young chefs when using any sharp tools or dealing with small pieces.

• Suggest they decorate the containers or bags with stickers or labels.

• Explain that the chocolate chips are optional and can be left out if desired.

13. VEGGIE STICKS WITH HUMMUS

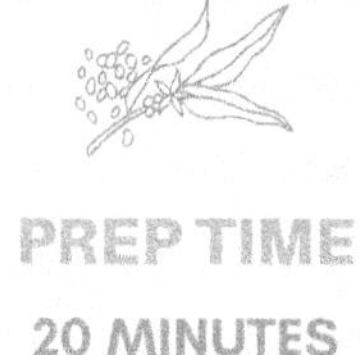 

PREP TIME
20 MINUTES

COOK TIME
30 MINUTES

INGREDIENTS:

• 1 cup baby carrots
• 1 cup cucumber slices
• 1 cup bell pepper strips (red, yellow, or orange)
• 1 cup cherry tomatoes
• 1 cup hummus (store•bought or homemade)

Tips for young chefs:

• Let the kids help wash and prepare the vegetables. Supervise them when using any sharp knives.

• Encourage them to try different types of vegetables, such as celery, broccoli, or zucchini.

• Suggest they make patterns or designs with the veggie sticks on the plate.

PROCEDURE:

1. Wash and prepare the vegetables:
   • Peel and slice the cucumber into sticks.
   • Cut the bell peppers into long, thin strips.
   • Leave the baby carrots whole or cut them in half if they are large.
   • Rinse the cherry tomatoes and leave them whole.

2. Arrange the prepared veggie sticks on a plate or platter.

3. Place the hummus in a small bowl in the center of the plate.

4. Encourage the young chefs to dip the veggie sticks into the hummus and enjoy!

• Offer a variety of hummus flavors, such as classic, roasted red pepper, or garlic.

• Remind them to wash their hands before and after handling the food.

• Discuss the importance of eating a variety of colorful vegetables.

This healthy and fun snack is a great way for young chefs to explore new foods and practice their kitchen skills.

14. POPCORN

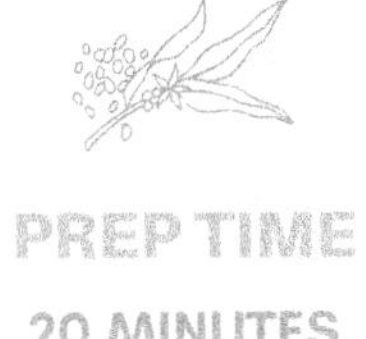

PREP TIME
20 MINUTES

COOK TIME
30 MINUTES

INGREDIENTS:

- 1/4 cup popcorn kernels
- 1•2 tablespoons vegetable or coconut oil
- Salt (optional)

Equipment:
- Large pot with a lid
- Popcorn popper (optional)

Tips for young chefs:

- Supervise young chefs closely when using the hot pot or popcorn popper.

- Encourage them to listen for the popping to slow down before removing from heat.

- Let them experiment with different seasonings, like garlic powder, chili powder, or parmesan cheese.

PROCEDURE:

1. If using a pot, add the oil to the pot and heat it over medium heat. If using a popcorn popper, follow the manufacturer's instructions.

2. Once the oil is hot, add the popcorn kernels in an even layer. Cover the pot with a lid.

3. Allow the kernels to start popping. Gently shake the pot or stir the popcorn popper to prevent burning.

4. Once the popping slows to 2•3 seconds between pops, remove the pot from the heat (or turn off the popcorn popper).

5. Carefully transfer the popped popcorn to a large bowl.

6. If desired, sprinkle the popcorn with a pinch of salt and toss to coat.

- Suggest they make patterns or designs with the popcorn in the bowl.

- Discuss food safety, such as washing hands before handling the popcorn.

- Offer small paper bags or containers for them to package the popcorn to share.

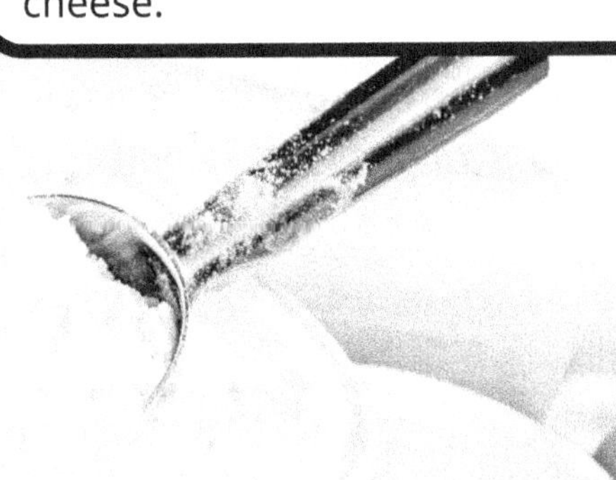

15. FRUIT KABOBS

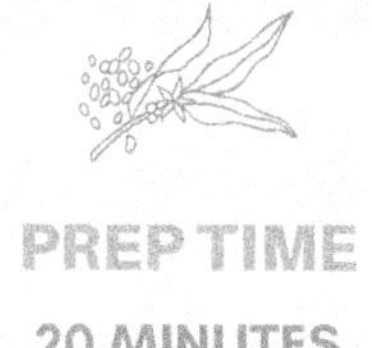

PREP TIME
20 MINUTES

COOK TIME
30 MINUTES

INGREDIENTS:

• Assorted fresh fruit (such as strawberries, grapes, pineapple, melon, kiwi, etc.)
• Wooden skewers or toothpicks

Tips for young chefs:

• Let the kids help wash and prepare the fruit. Supervise them when using any sharp knives.

• Encourage them to choose a variety of different colored fruits to make the kabobs look more appealing.

• Suggest they get creative with the fruit combinations and patterns on the skewers.

• Remind them to be gentle when threading the fruit to avoid breaking it.

PROCEDURE:

1. Wash and prepare the fruit:
   • Cut larger fruits, like pineapple or melon, into bite•sized pieces.
   • Leave smaller fruits, like grapes or berries, whole.

2. Carefully thread the fruit pieces onto the wooden skewers or toothpicks, creating a colorful pattern.

3. Arrange the fruit kabobs on a plate or platter.

• Discuss the importance of eating a rainbow of fruits and vegetables.

• Emphasize food safety, such as washing hands before handling the fruit.

• Ask an adult for help with any sharp tools or skewers.

• Offer a small bowl of yogurt or honey for dipping, if desired.

These colorful and healthy fruit kabobs are a fun and interactive snack for young chefs to make and enjoy.

16. CHEESE AND CRACKERS

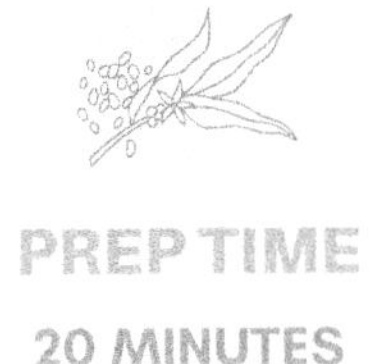 

PREP TIME
20 MINUTES

COOK TIME
30 MINUTES

INGREDIENTS:

• Assorted crackers (such as whole grain, wheat, or rice crackers)
• Sliced or cubed cheese (such as cheddar, gouda, or swiss)
• Optional toppings: grapes, apple slices, nuts, dried fruit

Tips for young chefs:

• Choose a variety of cracker types and cheese flavors for more interest.

• Cut the cheese into fun shapes using cookie cutters.

• Arrange the crackers and cheese in a creative pattern on the plate.

• Add a small bowl of olives, pickles, or other savory toppings for extra flavor.

PROCEDURE:

1. Arrange the crackers on a plate or platter.

2. Place the sliced or cubed cheese on the crackers.

3. If desired, add any additional toppings like grapes, apple slices, nuts, or dried fruit.

• Encourage kids to experiment with different cracker and cheese combinations.

• Remind young chefs to wash their hands before handling the food.

• Ask an adult for help with any sharp knives or tools needed.

This simple cheese and crackers snack is a great way for young chefs to get creative in the kitchen. Enjoy!

17. MINI QUESADILLAS

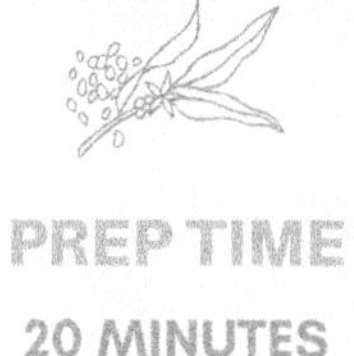

PREP TIME
20 MINUTES

COOK TIME
30 MINUTES

INGREDIENTS:

• 8 small flour or corn tortillas
• 1 cup shredded cheese (such as cheddar or Monterey Jack)
• Optional fillings: diced chicken, black beans, diced bell peppers, spinach, etc.

Tips for young chefs:

• Let the kids help measure and sprinkle the cheese and any other fillings.

• Encourage them to get creative with different ingredient combinations.

• Supervise them when using the hot pan or griddle.

• Remind them to be careful when cutting the quesadillas in half.

PROCEDURE:

1. Lay 4 of the tortillas on a clean, flat surface.

2. Sprinkle about 2•3 tablespoons of shredded cheese onto each tortilla, leaving a small border around the edges.

3. If using any additional fillings, place a small amount of the desired ingredients on top of the cheese.

4. Top each filled tortilla with another tortilla to create a mini quesadilla.

5. Heat a non•stick skillet or griddle over medium heat.

6. Carefully place the mini quesadillas in the hot pan and cook for 2•3 minutes per side, or until the tortillas are lightly golden and the cheese is melted.

7. Remove the quesadillas from the pan and cut each one in half to serve.

These mini quesadillas are a fun and easy snack for young chefs to make and enjoy!

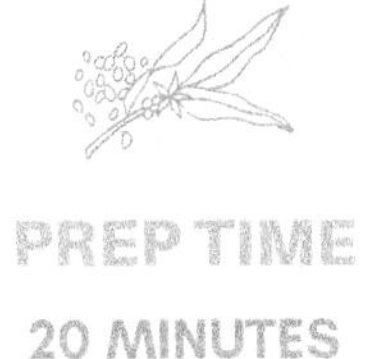

18. HOMEMADE GUACAMOLE AND CHIPS

PREP TIME
20 MINUTES

COOK TIME
30 MINUTES

INGREDIENTS :

Guacamole:
• 2 ripe avocados, halved and pitted
• 1 tablespoon lime juice
• 1 tablespoon diced onion
• 1 tablespoon diced tomato
• 1 teaspoon minced garlic
• 1/4 teaspoon salt

Chips:
• 8•10 corn tortillas, cut into triangles
• 2 tablespoons vegetable or olive oil
• 1/2 teaspoon salt

PROCEDURE :

Guacamole:
1. Scoop the avocado flesh into a bowl and mash it with a fork or potato masher.
2. Add the lime juice, onion, tomato, garlic, and salt. Stir to combine.
3. Taste and adjust seasoning as needed.

Chips:
1. Preheat the oven to 400°F (200°C).
2. Arrange the tortilla triangles in a single layer on a baking sheet.
3. Drizzle the oil over the chips and sprinkle with salt. Toss to coat evenly.
4. Bake for 8•10 minutes, flipping halfway, until the chips are crispy and lightly golden.

Tips for young chefs:
• Let the kids help mash the avocado and mix the guacamole ingredients.
• Supervise them when using a knife to cut the tortillas.
• Encourage them to experiment with different mix•in ideas, like jalapeño or cilantro.
• Discuss food safety, such as washing hands before handling the food.
• Ask an adult for help with the hot oven when baking the chips.
• Serve the guacamole and chips together for a delicious and healthy snack.

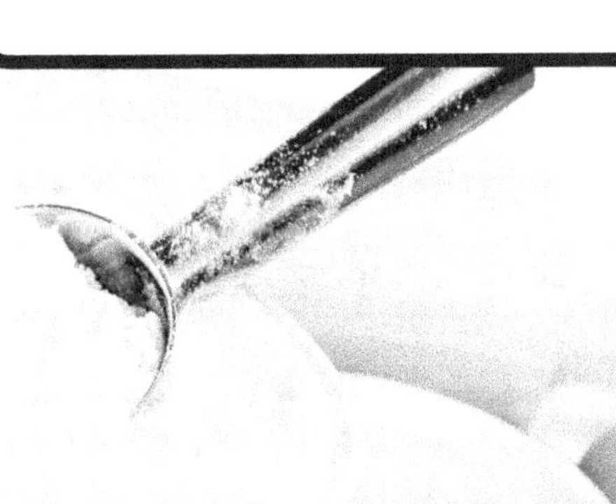

19. ANTS ON A LOG (CELERY WITH PEANUT BUTTER AND RAISINS)

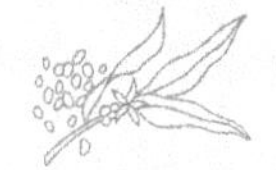 

PREP TIME
20 MINUTES

COOK TIME
30 MINUTES

INGREDIENTS:

- 3•4 celery stalks, cut into 3•4 inch pieces
- 2•3 tablespoons peanut butter
- 2•3 tablespoons raisins

This simple and fun snack is a great way for young chefs to practice their kitchen skills and explore new flavors. Enjoy your "Ants on a Log"!

PROCEDURE:

1. Wash the celery stalks and pat them dry.

2. Using a butter knife or spoon, spread a thin layer of peanut butter into the groove of each celery stick.

3. Gently press raisins into the peanut butter, spacing them out to look like "ants" on a log.

Tips for young chefs:

- Let the kids help wash and prepare the celery. Supervise them when using any knives.

- Encourage them to be creative with the placement of the raisins.

- Suggest they try different nut butters, like almond or cashew butter, instead of peanut butter.

- Offer other toppings like dried cranberries, mini chocolate chips, or chopped nuts.

- Discuss the importance of eating a variety of healthy snacks with protein, fiber, and nutrients.

- Remind them to wash their hands before and after handling the food.

20. SMOOTHIES

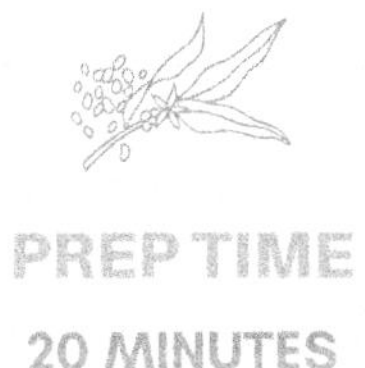

PREP TIME
20 MINUTES

COOK TIME
30 MINUTES

INGREDIENTS :

• 1 cup milk or non•dairy milk (such as almond, soy, or oat milk)
• 1 cup frozen fruit (such as strawberries, bananas, mango, or pineapple)
• 1/2 cup plain yogurt (optional)
• 1 tablespoon honey or maple syrup (optional)

Tips for young chefs:

• Let the kids help measure and add the ingredients to the blender.

• Encourage them to experiment with different fruit combinations.

PROCEDURE :

1. Add the milk, frozen fruit, yogurt (if using), and honey or maple syrup (if using) to a blender.

2. Blend the ingredients on high speed until the mixture is smooth and creamy, about 1•2 minutes.

3. Pour the smoothie into a glass or reusable cup.

4. Enjoy your delicious homemade smoothie!

• Suggest they try adding spinach, kale, or peanut butter for extra nutrition.

• Remind them to hold the blender lid firmly when blending to prevent spills.

• Supervise young chefs when using the blender, as the blades can be sharp.

• Discuss the importance of a balanced, healthy diet with fruits and vegetables.

• Offer small cups or straws for the kids to enjoy their smoothies.

Smoothies are a fun and nutritious snack or breakfast that young chefs can easily make themselves. Enjoy!

21. GRILLED CHEESE SANDWICHES

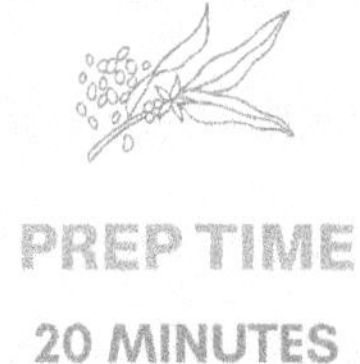

PREP TIME
20 MINUTES

COOK TIME
30 MINUTES

INGREDIENTS:

• 4 slices of bread (such as white, whole wheat, or sourdough)
• 2 slices of cheese (such as cheddar, American, or Swiss)
• 2 tablespoons butter or margarine

Tips for young chefs:

• Let the kids help assemble the sandwiches by placing the cheese and closing them up.
• Supervise them when using the hot pan or griddle.
• Encourage them to experiment with different types of bread and cheese.
• Suggest they add other fillings like tomato, ham, or bacon (with adult supervision).
• Remind them to wash their hands before and after handling the food.
• Offer a small bowl of tomato

PROCEDURE:

1. Lay the 4 slices of bread on a clean, flat surface.

2. Place one slice of cheese on 2 of the bread slices.

3. Top each cheese•topped slice with another slice of bread to create 2 sandwiches.

4. Heat a skillet or griddle over medium heat and add the butter or margarine.

5. Carefully place the sandwiches in the hot pan and cook for 2•3 minutes per side, or until the bread is golden brown and the cheese is melted.

6. Use a spatula to flip the sandwiches and cook the other side.

7. Remove the grilled cheese sandwiches from the pan and let them cool for a minute before serving.

Grilled cheese sandwiches are a classic and easy•to•make dish that young chefs will love!

22. TOMATO SOUP

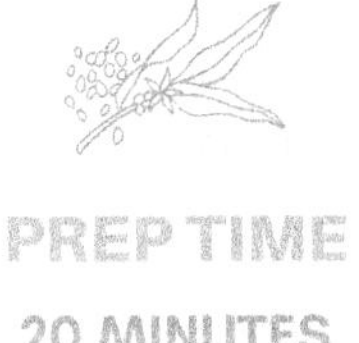 

PREP TIME
20 MINUTES

COOK TIME
30 MINUTES

INGREDIENTS:

- 1 (15 oz) can of diced tomatoes
- 1 cup of chicken or vegetable broth
- 1 tablespoon of butter or olive oil
- 1 tablespoon of sugar (optional)
- Salt and pepper to taste

Tips for young chefs:

- Let the kids help measure and pour the ingredients into the saucepan.

- Supervise them when using the blender or immersion blender, as the blades can be sharp.

- Encourage them to experiment with different toppings, like croutons, shredded cheese, or fresh basil.

PROCEDURE:

1. In a medium saucepan, combine the canned diced tomatoes and the broth.

2. Place the saucepan over medium heat and bring the mixture to a gentle simmer.

3. Add the butter or olive oil and stir until the butter is melted.

4. If desired, stir in the sugar to balance the acidity of the tomatoes.

5. Season with a pinch of salt and pepper to taste.

6. Carefully use a blender or immersion blender to puree the soup until smooth.

7. Return the pureed soup to the saucepan and heat through, stirring occasionally.

8. Ladle the warm tomato soup into bowls and serve.

This comforting tomato soup is a great way for young chefs to learn about making a simple, homemade meal.

23. CHICKEN SALAD WRAPS

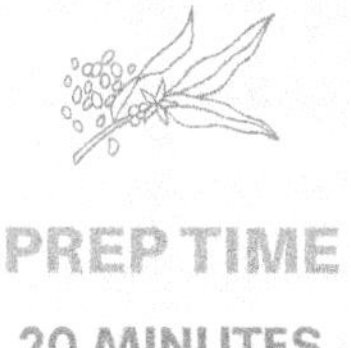 

INGREDIENTS:

- 2 cups cooked, shredded chicken
- 1/4 cup mayonnaise
- 1 tablespoon Dijon mustard
- 1 tablespoon lemon juice
- 1/4 cup diced celery
- 2 tablespoons diced onion (optional)
- Salt and pepper to taste
- 4•6 whole wheat tortillas or wraps

This easy and portable chicken salad wrap is a great option for a healthy lunch or snack that young chefs can help prepare.

PROCEDURE:

1. In a medium bowl, mix together the shredded chicken, mayonnaise, Dijon mustard, lemon juice, celery, and onion (if using). Season with salt and pepper to taste.

2. Lay the tortillas or wraps on a clean surface. Scoop about 1/2 cup of the chicken salad mixture onto the center of each wrap.

3. Fold the bottom of the wrap up over the filling, then fold in the sides and continue rolling up tightly to create a wrap.

4. Cut the wraps in half diagonally, if desired, and serve.

Tips for young chefs:

- Let the kids help measure and mix the ingredients for the chicken salad.

- Encourage them to use a fork or their hands to shred the cooked chicken.

- Suggest they add other crunchy veggies like carrots or bell peppers.

- Remind them to wash their hands before and after handling the food.

24. TUNA SALAD

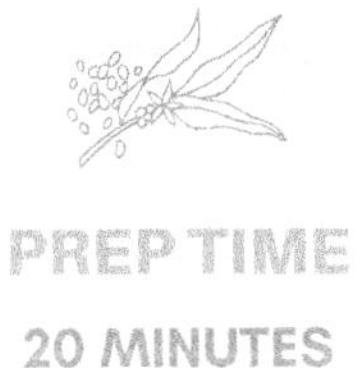

PREP TIME
20 MINUTES

COOK TIME
30 MINUTES

INGREDIENTS:

- 1 (5 oz) can of tuna, drained
- 2 tablespoons mayonnaise
- 1 tablespoon diced celery
- 1 tablespoon diced onion (optional)
- 1 teaspoon lemon juice
- Salt and pepper to taste

This simple tuna salad is a great protein•packed option for a healthy snack or light meal that young chefs can help prepare.

PROCEDURE:

1. In a medium bowl, use a fork to flake the drained tuna into small pieces.

2. Add the mayonnaise, diced celery, diced onion (if using), and lemon juice. Stir to combine.

3. Season the tuna salad with a pinch of salt and pepper to taste.

4. Serve the tuna salad on crackers, bread, or lettuce leaves.

Tips for young chefs:

- Let the kids help measure and mix the ingredients in the bowl.
- Encourage them to use a fork to gently flake the tuna.
- Suggest they add other crunchy veggies like diced carrot or bell pepper.
- Remind them to wash their hands before and after handling the food.
- Supervise young chefs when using any sharp knives or tools.
- Offer small plates or bowls for them to serve the tuna salad.
- Discuss the importance of food safety and proper food handling.

25. HOMEMADE PIZZA

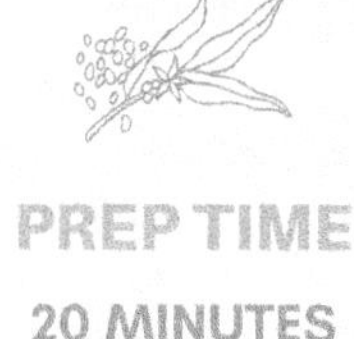 

PREP TIME
20 MINUTES

COOK TIME
30 MINUTES

INGREDIENTS:

- 1 pre•made pizza crust or dough
- 1/2 cup pizza sauce
- 1 cup shredded mozzarella cheese
- Assorted toppings (such as pepperoni, mushrooms, bell peppers, onions)

Tips for young chefs:

- Let the kids help roll or stretch out the dough (if using).

- Encourage them to get creative with the toppings, such as arranging the pepperoni in a pattern.

- Supervise them when using the oven, as it can be hot.

PROCEDURE:

1. Preheat the oven to 400°F (200°C).

2. If using pre•made dough, roll or stretch it out to fit your pizza pan or baking sheet. If using a pre•made crust, skip this step.

3. Spread the pizza sauce evenly over the crust, leaving a small border around the edges.

4. Sprinkle the shredded mozzarella cheese over the sauce.

5. Add your desired toppings, arranging them evenly over the cheese.

6. Bake the pizza in the preheated oven for 12•15 minutes, or until the crust is golden brown and the cheese is melted and bubbly.

7. Remove the pizza from the oven and let it cool for a few minutes before slicing and serving.

Homemade pizza is a fun and interactive way for young chefs to get involved in the kitchen and create a delicious meal.

26. PASTA SALAD

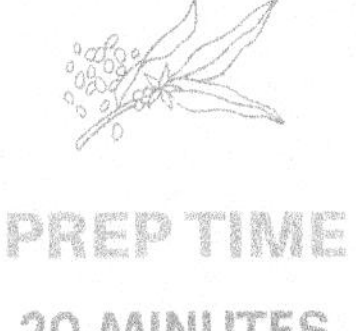

PREP TIME
20 MINUTES

COOK TIME
30 MINUTES

INGREDIENTS:

- 2 cups cooked and cooled pasta (such as rotini, penne, or farfalle)
- 1/2 cup diced cucumber
- 1/2 cup diced cherry tomatoes
- 1/4 cup diced bell pepper
- 2 tablespoons Italian dressing
- 1 tablespoon grated Parmesan cheese (optional)
- Salt and pepper to taste

Tips for young chefs:

- Let the kids help measure and add the ingredients to the bowl.

- Encourage them to choose their favorite pasta shapes and vegetables.

- Suggest they use different colored bell peppers for a more vibrant salad.

PROCEDURE:

1. In a large bowl, combine the cooked and cooled pasta, diced cucumber, tomatoes, and bell pepper.

2. Add the Italian dressing and toss gently to coat the pasta and vegetables.

3. If desired, sprinkle the Parmesan cheese over the top.

4. Season with a pinch of salt and pepper to taste.

5. Chill the pasta salad in the refrigerator for at least 30 minutes before serving.

- Supervise young chefs when using any sharp knives or tools.

- Offer small bowls or plates for them to serve the pasta salad.

- Discuss the importance of letting the pasta cool completely before assembling the salad.

- Remind them to wash their hands before and after handling the food.

This easy and customizable pasta salad is a great way for young chefs to learn about combining different flavors and textures in a healthy dish.

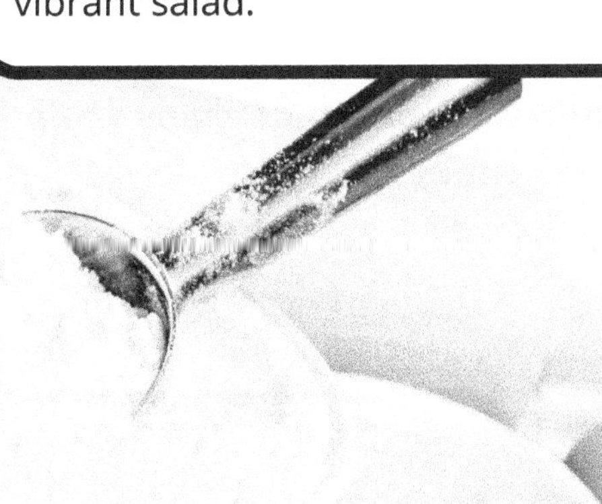

27. MAC AND CHEESE

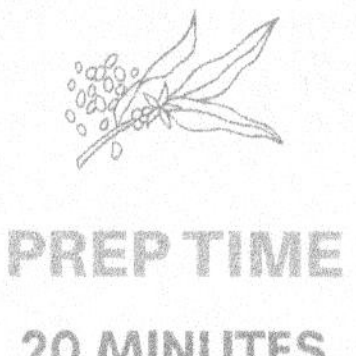

PREP TIME
20 MINUTES

COOK TIME
30 MINUTES

INGREDIENTS:

- 8 oz elbow macaroni
- 2 tablespoons butter
- 2 tablespoons all•purpose flour
- 2 cups milk
- 2 cups shredded cheddar cheese
- 1/4 teaspoon salt
- 1/8 teaspoon black pepper

Tips for young chefs:

- Let the kids help measure and add the ingredients to the pot and saucepan.

- Supervise them when working with the hot stove and saucepan.

- Encourage them to experiment with different types of cheese or add•ins like diced ham or peas.

- Remind them to wash their hands before and after handling the food.

PROCEDURE:

1. Bring a large pot of salted water to a boil. Cook the macaroni according to the package instructions until al dente. Drain and set aside.

2. In a medium saucepan, melt the butter over medium heat. Whisk in the flour and cook for 1•2 minutes, stirring constantly, to make a roux.

3. Gradually whisk in the milk, a little at a time, until the sauce is smooth and thickened, about 5 minutes.

4. Remove the saucepan from the heat and stir in the shredded cheddar cheese until it's melted and the sauce is smooth. Season with salt and pepper.

5. Add the cooked macaroni to the cheese sauce and stir to combine.

6. Serve the mac and cheese warm, with additional toppings like breadcrumbs or chopped parsley, if desired.

This classic homemade mac and cheese is a comforting and kid•friendly dish that young chefs will enjoy making and eating.

28. CHICKEN TENDERS

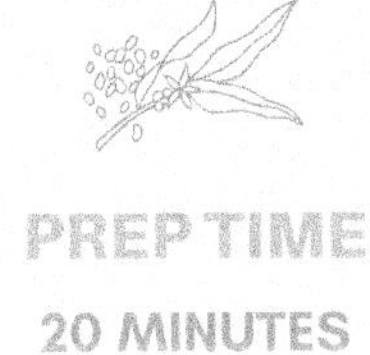

PREP TIME
20 MINUTES

COOK TIME
30 MINUTES

INGREDIENTS:

- 1 lb boneless, skinless chicken breasts, cut into strips
- 1 cup all•purpose flour
- 2 eggs, beaten
- 1 cup breadcrumbs or panko
- 1/2 teaspoon salt
- 1/4 teaspoon black pepper
- Vegetable oil for frying

Tips for young chefs:

- Let the kids help with the breading process, dipping the chicken in the flour, eggs, and breadcrumbs.

- Supervise them when working with the hot oil and frying the chicken.

- Encourage them to experiment with different seasoning blends or dipping sauces.

PROCEDURE:

1. Set up a breading station with three shallow dishes: one with the flour, one with the beaten eggs, and one with the breadcrumbs or panko.

2. Season the chicken strips with salt and pepper.

3. Dredge the chicken strips in the flour, dip them in the beaten eggs, and then coat them in the breadcrumbs or panko, pressing gently to help the coating adhere.

4. In a large skillet, heat about 1/2 inch of vegetable oil over medium•high heat.

5. Carefully add the breaded chicken tenders to the hot oil and fry for 2•3 minutes per side, or until golden brown and cooked through.

6. Transfer the fried chicken tenders to a paper towel•lined plate to drain any excess oil.

7. Serve the chicken tenders warm, with your favorite dipping sauces on the side.

These homemade chicken tenders are a delicious and kid•friendly meal that young chefs can help prepare.

29. TURKEY AND CHEESE ROLL•UPS

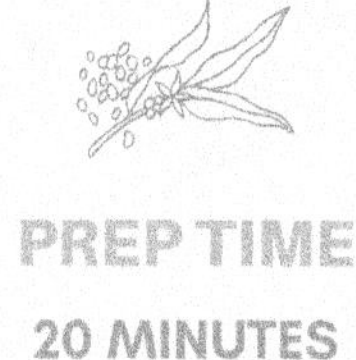

PREP TIME
20 MINUTES

COOK TIME
30 MINUTES

INGREDIENTS:

- 4 slices of deli turkey
- 4 slices of cheese (such as cheddar, Swiss, or provolone)
- 4 whole wheat tortillas or wraps

Tips for young chefs:

- Let the kids help assemble the roll•ups by placing the cheese and turkey.

- Encourage them to be gentle when rolling up the tortillas to prevent tearing.

- Suggest they try different combinations of meats and cheeses.

- Remind them to wash their hands before and after handling the food.

PROCEDURE:

1. Lay the tortillas or wraps on a clean, flat surface.

2. Place one slice of cheese on each tortilla, leaving a small border around the edges.

3. Top the cheese with one slice of deli turkey.

4. Carefully roll up the tortilla, starting from one side and rolling tightly to the other side.

5. Use a toothpick or small skewer to secure the roll•up, if needed.

6. Repeat steps 2•5 with the remaining tortillas, cheese, and turkey. Slice the roll•ups in half diagonally, if desired, and serve.

- Supervise young chefs when using any sharp tools, like toothpicks or skewers.

- Offer small plates or napkins for them to enjoy their roll•ups.

- Discuss the importance of food safety and proper food handling.

These simple and portable turkey and cheese roll•ups are a great option for a healthy snack or lunch that young chefs can help prepare.

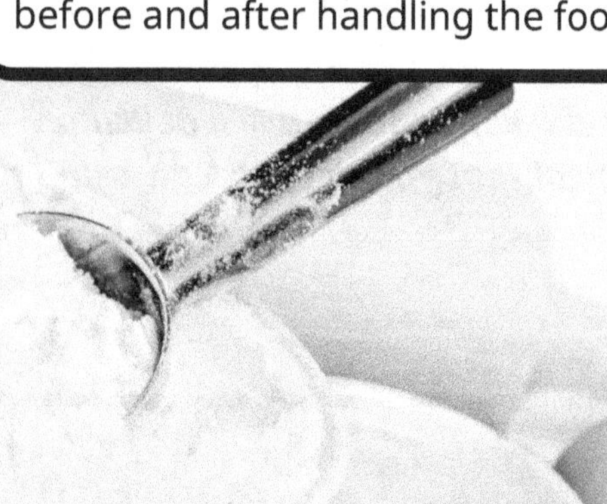

30. MINI BAGEL PIZZAS

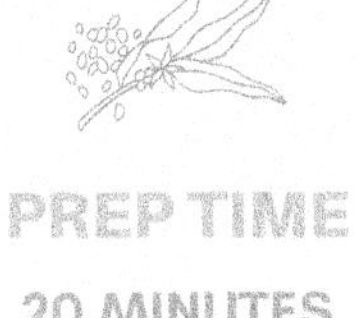

PREP TIME
20 MINUTES

COOK TIME
30 MINUTES

INGREDIENTS:

• 4 mini bagels, split in half
• 1/2 cup pizza sauce
• 1 cup shredded mozzarella cheese
• Assorted toppings (such as pepperoni, mushrooms, bell peppers, olives)

Tips for young chefs:

• Let the kids help assemble the mini pizzas by adding the sauce, cheese, and toppings.

• Encourage them to get creative with different topping combinations.

• Supervise them when using the oven, as it can be hot.

• Remind them to wash their hands before and after handling the food.

PROCEDURE:

1. Preheat the oven to 400°F (200°C).

2. Place the bagel halves on a baking sheet or oven•safe plate.

3. Spread a spoonful of pizza sauce onto each bagel half, leaving a small border around the edges.

4. Sprinkle the shredded mozzarella cheese over the sauce.

5. Add your desired toppings, such as pepperoni, mushrooms, bell peppers, or olives.

6. Bake the mini bagel pizzas in the preheated oven for 8•10 minutes, or until the cheese is melted and bubbly.

7. Remove the pizzas from the oven and let them cool for a minute before serving.

These mini bagel pizzas are a fun and easy way for young chefs to make their own personalized pizzas.

31. SPAGHETTI AND MEATBALLS

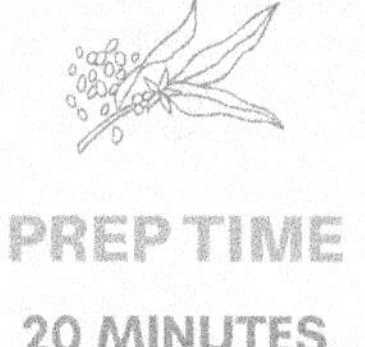

INGREDIENTS :

- 1 lb ground beef
- 1/2 cup breadcrumbs
- 1/4 cup grated Parmesan cheese
- 1 egg
- 1 tsp dried oregano
- 1/2 tsp garlic powder
- Salt and pepper to taste
- 8 oz spaghetti pasta
- 1 jar (24 oz) marinara sauce

This recipe is easy for young chefs to follow and makes a delicious, classic Italian•American dish. Encourage them to get involved in the meatball rolling and sauce simmering steps.

PROCEDURE :

1. In a medium bowl, mix together the ground beef, breadcrumbs, Parmesan cheese, egg, oregano, garlic powder, salt, and pepper until well combined.

2. Roll the mixture into small, bite•sized meatballs, about 1•inch in size.

3. In a large pot, bring salted water to a boil. Add the spaghetti and cook according to package instructions until al dente.

4. In a large skillet, gently place the meatballs and cook over medium heat, turning occasionally, until browned on all sides and cooked through, about 10•12 minutes.

5. Pour the marinara sauce into the skillet with the meatballs and stir to coat. Simmer for 5•10 minutes to allow the flavors to blend.

6. Drain the cooked spaghetti and transfer to a serving dish. Top with the meatballs and sauce.

7. Serve hot, with additional Parmesan cheese and fresh basil leaves if desired.

32. TACOS

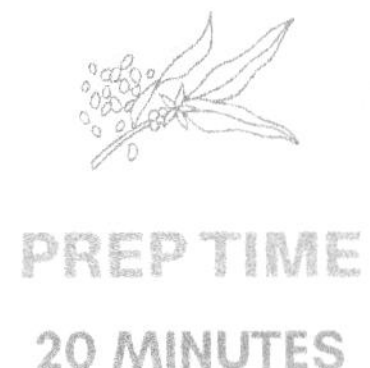 

PREP TIME
20 MINUTES

COOK TIME
30 MINUTES

INGREDIENTS:

- 1 lb ground beef or turkey
- 1 packet taco seasoning
- 8•10 taco shells or soft tortillas
- 1 cup shredded lettuce
- 1 cup diced tomatoes
- 1 cup shredded cheddar cheese
- Sour cream (optional)
- Salsa (optional)

Tips for young chefs:
• Let the kids help measure and add the ingredients to the skillet.

• Supervise them when using the stove, as it can be hot.

• Encourage them to get creative with their taco toppings.

• Remind them to wash their hands before and after handling the food.

PROCEDURE:

1. In a skillet, cook the ground beef or turkey over medium heat until browned and crumbled. Drain any excess fat.

2. Stir in the taco seasoning and the amount of water specified on the seasoning packet. Simmer for 5•7 minutes, stirring occasionally, until the sauce has thickened.

3. Warm the taco shells or tortillas according to the package instructions.

4. To assemble the tacos, place a spoonful of the seasoned ground meat into each taco shell or tortilla.

5. Top the meat with shredded lettuce, diced tomatoes, and shredded cheese.

6. If desired, add a dollop of sour cream and/or salsa.

7. Serve the tacos immediately.

Tacos are a fun and interactive meal that young chefs can help prepare and customize to their liking.

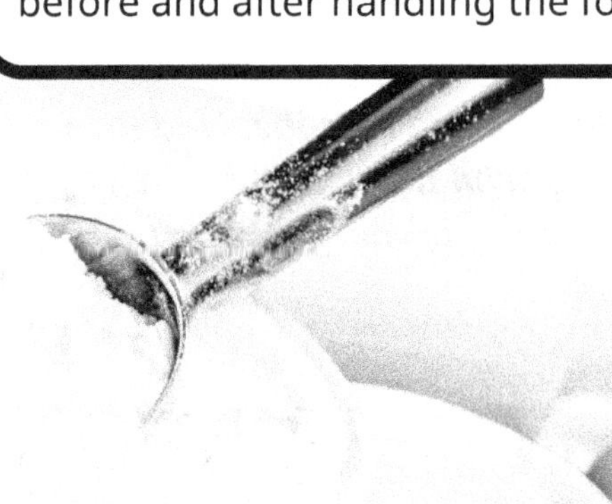

33. STIR•FRIED VEGGIES AND RICE

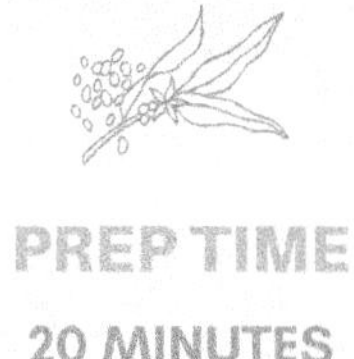 

INGREDIENTS:

- 1 cup uncooked white or brown rice
- 2 tablespoons vegetable oil
- 1 cup broccoli florets
- 1 cup sliced carrots
- 1 cup sliced mushrooms
- 1 cup snow peas or snap peas
- 2 cloves garlic, minced
- 2 tablespoons soy sauce
- 1 teaspoon sesame oil (optional)
- Salt and pepper to taste

Tips for young chefs:

- Let them help measure and add the ingredients.

- Demonstrate how to safely use a knife to slice the vegetables.

- Encourage them to try different vegetable combinations.

PROCEDURE:

1. Cook the rice according to package instructions. Set aside.

2. In a large skillet or wok, heat the vegetable oil over medium•high heat.

3. Add the broccoli, carrots, mushrooms, and snow/snap peas. Stir•fry for 5•7 minutes, until the vegetables are tender•crisp.

4. Add the minced garlic and stir•fry for 1 minute more, until fragrant.

5. Pour in the soy sauce and sesame oil (if using). Stir to coat the vegetables.

6. Add the cooked rice to the skillet and toss everything together until well combined and heated through.

7. Season with salt and pepper to taste.

8. Serve the stir•fried veggies and rice hot.

This dish is a great way to get kids involved in cooking a healthy, flavorful meal. Adjust the spices and vegetables to suit your family's tastes.

34. BAKED ZITI

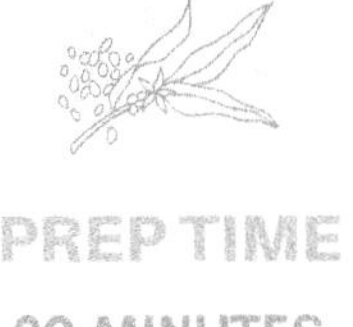

PREP TIME
20 MINUTES

COOK TIME
30 MINUTES

INGREDIENTS:

- 8 oz ziti or penne pasta
- 1 lb ground beef or Italian sausage
- 1 jar (24 oz) marinara sauce
- 1 cup ricotta cheese
- 1 cup shredded mozzarella cheese
- 1/4 cup grated Parmesan cheese
- 1 egg
- 1/4 cup chopped fresh basil (optional)
- Salt and pepper to taste

Tips for young chefs:

- Let the kids help measure and mix the ingredients in the bowl.

- Supervise them when using the stove or oven, as they can be hot.

PROCEDURE:

1. Preheat the oven to 375°F (190°C).

2. Cook the pasta according to the package instructions. Drain and set aside.

3. In a skillet, cook the ground beef or sausage over medium heat until browned and crumbled. Drain any excess fat.

4. In a large bowl, mix the cooked pasta, browned meat, marinara sauce, ricotta cheese, 1/2 cup of the mozzarella cheese, Parmesan cheese, egg, and basil (if using). Season with salt and pepper.

5. Spread the pasta mixture into a 9x13 inch baking dish. Top with the remaining 1/2 cup of mozzarella cheese.

6. Bake for 25•30 minutes, or until the cheese is melted and bubbly.

7. Let the baked ziti cool for 5 minutes before serving.

This cheesy and comforting baked ziti is a great dish for young chefs to help prepare.

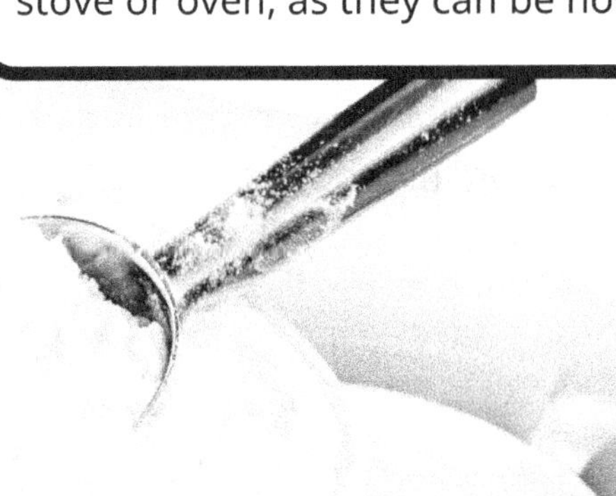

35. CHICKEN ALFREDO

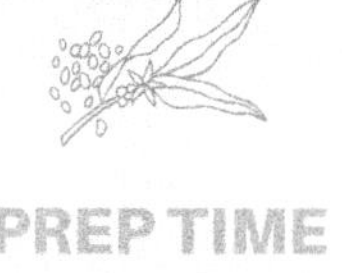

PREP TIME
20 MINUTES

COOK TIME
30 MINUTES

INGREDIENTS:

• 8 oz fettuccine pasta
• 2 boneless, skinless chicken breasts
• 2 tablespoons olive oil
• 1/2 cup heavy cream
• 1/2 cup grated Parmesan cheese
• 2 cloves garlic, minced
• 2 tablespoons butter
• Salt and pepper to taste
• Chopped parsley for garnish (optional)

Tips for young chefs:
• Let them help measure and add the ingredients.

• Demonstrate how to safely cook the chicken and boil the pasta.

• Encourage them to taste the sauce and suggest seasonings.

• Discuss the importance of food safety when handling raw chicken.

PROCEDURE:

1. Bring a large pot of salted water to a boil. Add the fettuccine and cook according to package instructions until al dente. Drain and set aside.

2. Season the chicken breasts with salt and pepper.

3. In a large skillet, heat the olive oil over medium•high heat. Add the chicken and cook for 5•7 minutes per side, until cooked through. Remove the chicken from the skillet and let it rest for a few minutes, then slice or shred it.

4. In the same skillet, reduce the heat to medium•low. Add the heavy cream, Parmesan cheese, and garlic. Whisk the mixture together and let it simmer for 2•3 minutes, until the sauce thickens slightly.

5. Add the cooked fettuccine and the sliced or shredded chicken to the skillet. Toss everything together until the pasta is evenly coated in the Alfredo sauce.

6. Remove the skillet from the heat and stir in the butter until it's melted and incorporated.

7. Serve the Chicken Alfredo immediately, garnished with chopped parsley if desired.

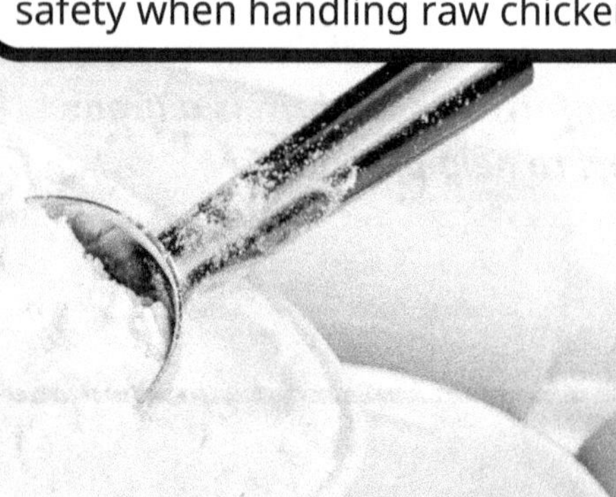

36. SLOPPY JOES

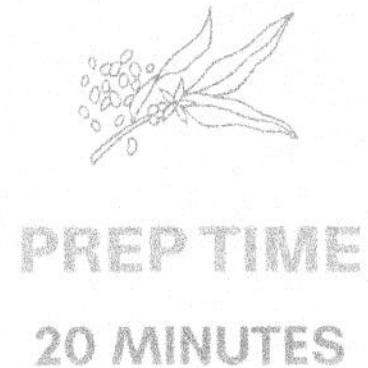 

INGREDIENTS :

- 1 lb ground beef
- 1 onion, diced
- 1 green bell pepper, diced
- 2 cloves garlic, minced
- 1 cup ketchup
- 2 tablespoons brown sugar
- 2 tablespoons Worcestershire sauce
- 1 teaspoon mustard powder
- 1/2 teaspoon chili powder
- Salt and pepper to taste
- 6•8 hamburger buns

Sloppy Joes are a classic, kid•friendly meal that's easy for young chefs to make. Serve with a side of carrot sticks, apple slices, or a simple salad for a well•rounded meal.

PROCEDURE :

1. In a large skillet over medium•high heat, cook the ground beef, onion, bell pepper, and garlic until the beef is browned and the vegetables are tender, about 5•7 minutes. Drain any excess fat.

2. Stir in the ketchup, brown sugar, Worcestershire sauce, mustard powder, and chili powder. Season with salt and pepper to taste.

3. Reduce the heat to low and let the sloppy joe mixture simmer for 10•15 minutes, stirring occasionally, until the flavors have melded and the sauce has thickened.

4. Spoon the sloppy joe mixture onto the hamburger buns and serve immediately.

Tips for young chefs:

- Let them help measure and add the ingredients.

- Demonstrate how to safely brown the ground beef and chop the vegetables.

- Encourage them to taste the mixture and suggest seasonings.

- Discuss the importance of food safety when handling raw meat.

37. STUFFED BELL PEPPERS

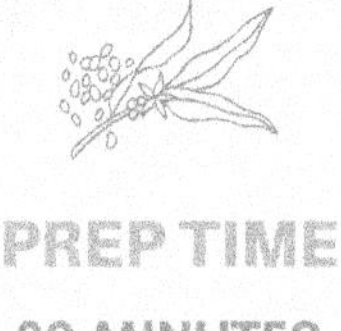

PREP TIME
20 MINUTES

COOK TIME
30 MINUTES

INGREDIENTS:

- 4 bell peppers (any color)
- 1 lb ground beef or ground turkey
- 1 cup cooked rice
- 1/2 cup diced onion
- 2 cloves garlic, minced
- 1 teaspoon dried oregano
- 1/2 teaspoon salt
- 1/4 teaspoon black pepper
- 1 cup shredded cheddar or mozzarella cheese

Tips for young chefs:

- Let them help measure and add the ingredients.

- Demonstrate how to safely cut the tops off the peppers and remove the seeds.

- Encourage them to taste the filling mixture and suggest seasonings.

PROCEDURE:

1. Preheat your oven to 375°F (190°C).

2. Cut the tops off the bell peppers and remove the seeds and membranes. Place the peppers in a baking dish.

3. In a large bowl, mix together the ground beef or turkey, cooked rice, onion, garlic, oregano, salt, and pepper until well combined.

4. Spoon the meat mixture evenly into the hollowed•out bell peppers.

5. Top each stuffed pepper with a sprinkle of shredded cheese.

6. Cover the baking dish with foil and bake for 30•35 minutes, or until the peppers are tender and the filling is cooked through.

7. Remove the foil and bake for an additional 5•10 minutes, or until the cheese is melted and lightly browned. Serve the Stuffed Bell Peppers hot.

Stuffed Bell Peppers are a fun, interactive dish that allows young chefs to get involved in the preparation. Serve with a side salad or roasted vegetables for a well•rounded meal.

38. CHICKEN PARMESAN

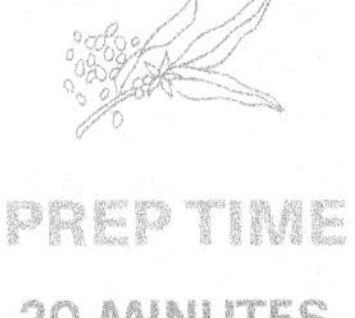

PREP TIME
20 MINUTES

COOK TIME
30 MINUTES

INGREDIENTS:

- 4 boneless, skinless chicken breasts
- 1 cup all•purpose flour
- 2 eggs, beaten
- 1 cup breadcrumbs
- 1/2 cup grated Parmesan cheese
- 1 teaspoon dried oregano
- 1/2 teaspoon garlic powder
- Salt and pepper to taste
- 1 jar (24 oz) marinara sauce
- 1 cup shredded mozzarella cheese

Chicken Parmesan is a classic, family•friendly dish that's easy for young chefs to make. The breading and melted cheese make it a crowd•pleaser.

PROCEDURE:

1. Preheat your oven to 400°F (200°C).

2. Place the chicken breasts between two sheets of plastic wrap or parchment paper and pound them to an even thickness, about 1/2 inch thick.

3. Set up three shallow dishes: one with the flour, one with the beaten eggs, and one with the breadcrumbs, Parmesan cheese, oregano, garlic powder, salt, and pepper mixed together.

4. Dredge the chicken breasts in the flour, dip them in the egg, and then coat them in the breadcrumb mixture, pressing gently to help it adhere.

5. Place the breaded chicken breasts in a baking dish or on a baking sheet lined with parchment paper. Bake the chicken for 20•25 minutes, or until it's cooked through and the breading is golden brown.

6. Pour the marinara sauce over the chicken and top with the shredded mozzarella cheese. Return the dish to the oven and bake for an additional 10•15 minutes, or until the cheese is melted and bubbly.

39. SHEPHERD'S PIE

PREP TIME
20 MINUTES

COOK TIME
30 MINUTES

INGREDIENTS:

- 1 lb ground beef or ground lamb
- 1 onion, diced
- 2 carrots, peeled and diced
- 2 cloves garlic, minced
- 1 tablespoon tomato paste
- 1 cup beef or chicken broth
- 1 teaspoon Worcestershire sauce
- 1 teaspoon dried thyme
- Salt and pepper to taste
- 3 cups mashed potatoes (about 4•5 medium potatoes)
- 1/2 cup shredded cheddar cheese

Shepherd's Pie is a comforting, family•friendly dish that's easy for young chefs to make. Serve with a side salad or steamed vegetables for a well•rounded meal.

PROCEDURE:

1. Preheat your oven to 375°F (190°C).

2. In a large skillet, cook the ground beef or lamb over medium•high heat, breaking it up with a wooden spoon, until browned, about 5•7 minutes. Drain any excess fat.

3. Add the diced onion and carrots to the skillet and cook for 5 minutes, until the vegetables are softened.

4. Stir in the minced garlic and tomato paste, and cook for 1 minute. Pour in the broth and Worcestershire sauce, and add the dried thyme. Season with salt and pepper to taste.

5. Bring the mixture to a simmer and let it cook for 10•15 minutes, or until the sauce has thickened. Transfer the meat and vegetable mixture to a 9x13•inch baking dish.

6. Spread the mashed potatoes evenly over the top of the meat mixture. Sprinkle the shredded cheddar cheese over the mashed potatoes.

7. Bake the Shepherd's Pie in the preheated oven for 25•30 minutes, or until the potatoes are lightly browned and the filling is bubbly. Let the Shepherd's Pie cool for 5•10 minutes before serving.

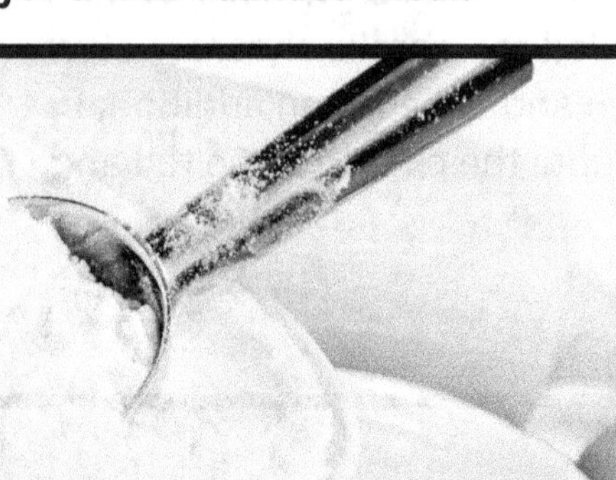

40. MEATLOAF

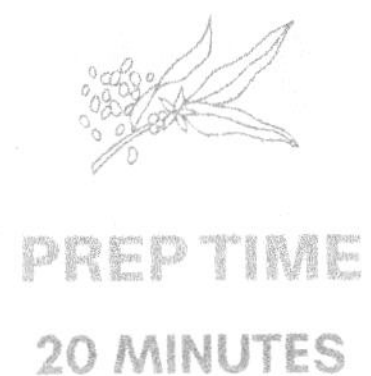

PREP TIME
20 MINUTES

COOK TIME
30 MINUTES

INGREDIENTS:

- 1 lb ground beef
- 1 cup breadcrumbs
- 1 egg
- 1/2 cup milk
- 1 onion, finely chopped
- 2 cloves garlic, minced
- 1 teaspoon dried oregano
- 1 teaspoon salt
- 1/2 teaspoon black pepper
- 1/2 cup ketchup or barbecue sauce (for topping)

Tips for young chefs:

- Let them help measure and add the ingredients.
- Demonstrate how to safely mix the meatloaf mixture with their hands.
- Encourage them to taste the mixture and suggest seasonings.
- Discuss the importance of food safety when handling raw meat.

PROCEDURE:

1. Preheat your oven to 375°F (190°C).

2. In a large bowl, combine the ground beef, breadcrumbs, egg, milk, onion, garlic, oregano, salt, and pepper. Mix everything together until well combined.

3. Grease a 9x5•inch loaf pan. Transfer the meatloaf mixture to the prepared pan, shaping it into a loaf.

4. Spread the ketchup or barbecue sauce evenly over the top of the meatloaf.

5. Bake the meatloaf in the preheated oven for 55•60 minutes, or until the internal temperature reaches 160°F (71°C).

6. Remove the meatloaf from the oven and let it rest for 5•10 minutes before slicing and serving.

Meatloaf is a classic, comforting dish that's easy for young chefs to make. Serve it with mashed potatoes, roasted vegetables, or a simple salad for a well•rounded meal.

41. GARLIC BREAD

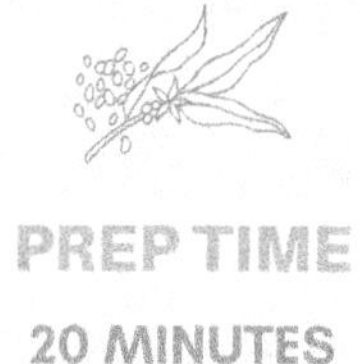

PREP TIME
20 MINUTES

COOK TIME
30 MINUTES

INGREDIENTS:

• 1 loaf of French or Italian bread, sliced in half lengthwise
• 1/2 cup (1 stick) unsalted butter, softened
• 3 cloves garlic, minced
• 1 teaspoon dried parsley
• 1/4 teaspoon salt

Tips for young chefs:

• Let them help measure and mix the garlic butter ingredients.

• Demonstrate how to safely use a knife to mince the garlic.

• Encourage them to taste the garlic butter and suggest adjustments.

• Discuss the importance of food safety when handling raw garlic.

PROCEDURE:

1. Preheat your oven to 400°F (200°C).

2. In a small bowl, mix together the softened butter, minced garlic, dried parsley, and salt until well combined.

3. Spread the garlic butter mixture evenly over the cut sides of the bread.

4. Place the bread, cut•side up, on a baking sheet or in a baking dish.

5. Bake the garlic bread in the preheated oven for 10•12 minutes, or until the bread is lightly toasted and the butter is melted.

6. Remove the garlic bread from the oven and let it cool for a few minutes.

7. Slice the garlic bread into pieces and serve warm.

Garlic Bread is a simple, flavorful side dish that's easy for young chefs to make. Serve it alongside pasta dishes, soups, or as a snack. Encourage kids to experiment with different herbs or cheese toppings to customize the recipe.

42. ROASTED VEGETABLES

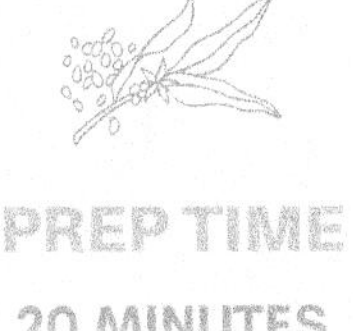

PREP TIME
20 MINUTES

COOK TIME
30 MINUTES

INGREDIENTS:

• 2 cups chopped vegetables (such as broccoli, cauliflower, carrots, zucchini, bell peppers)
• 2 tablespoons olive oil
• 1 teaspoon dried herbs (such as oregano, thyme, or rosemary)
• Salt and pepper to taste

Roasted Vegetables are a simple, healthy, and versatile side dish that's easy for young chefs to prepare. The hands•on nature of this recipe allows kids to get involved in the cooking process. Serve the roasted vegetables as a side dish or incorporate them into other meals, such as pasta or rice bowls.

PROCEDURE:

1. Preheat your oven to 400°F (200°C).

2. In a large bowl, toss the chopped vegetables with the olive oil, dried herbs, salt, and pepper until they are evenly coated.

3. Spread the seasoned vegetables in a single layer on a baking sheet or in a roasting pan.

4. Roast the vegetables in the preheated oven for 20•25 minutes, or until they are tender and lightly browned, stirring halfway through.

5. Remove the roasted vegetables from the oven and serve hot.

Tips for young chefs:

• Let them help wash, chop, and toss the vegetables.
• Encourage them to choose their favorite vegetables to include.
• Demonstrate how to safely use a knife to chop the vegetables.
• Discuss the importance of eating a variety of colorful vegetables.
• Suggest they try different herb and seasoning combinations

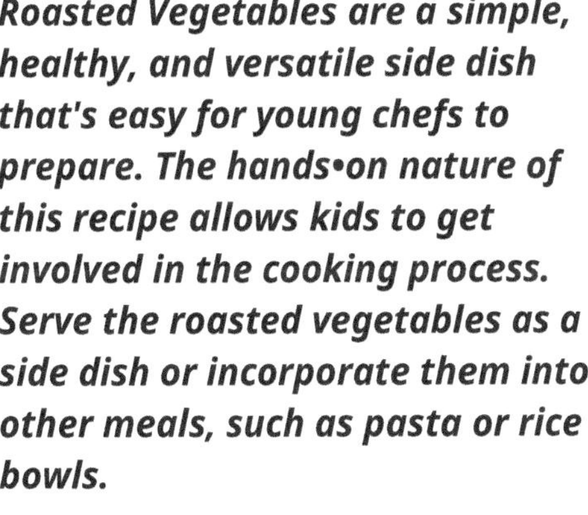

43. MASHED POTATOES

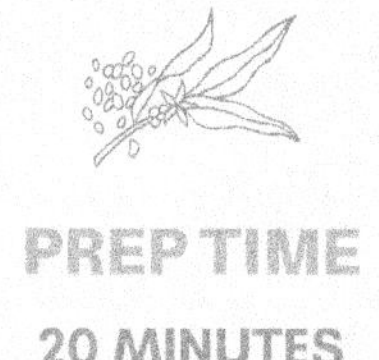 

PREP TIME
20 MINUTES

COOK TIME
30 MINUTES

INGREDIENTS :

• 3 lbs Russet or Yukon Gold potatoes, peeled and cut into 1•inch cubes
• 1/2 cup milk
• 4 tablespoons butter
• 1 teaspoon salt
• 1/4 teaspoon black pepper

Tips for young chefs:

• Let them help peel and cube the potatoes.

• Demonstrate how to safely use a potato masher or hand mixer.

• Encourage them to taste the potatoes and suggest seasonings.

• Discuss the importance of food safety when handling hot items.

PROCEDURE :

1. Place the cubed potatoes in a large pot and cover with cold water.

2. Bring the water to a boil over high heat, then reduce the heat to medium•low and simmer for 15•20 minutes, or until the potatoes are very tender when pierced with a fork.

3. Drain the potatoes in a colander and return them to the pot.

4. Add the milk, butter, salt, and pepper to the pot with the potatoes.

5. Using a potato masher or an electric hand mixer, mash the potatoes until they are smooth and creamy, with no lumps.

6. Taste the mashed potatoes and adjust the seasoning with additional salt and pepper if desired. Serve the mashed potatoes hot.

Mashed potatoes are a classic, comforting side dish that's easy for young chefs to make. Serve them alongside roasted meats, stews, or as a base for other dishes. Encourage kids to get creative by adding their favorite mix•ins, such as cheese, chives, or roasted garlic.

44. COLESLAW

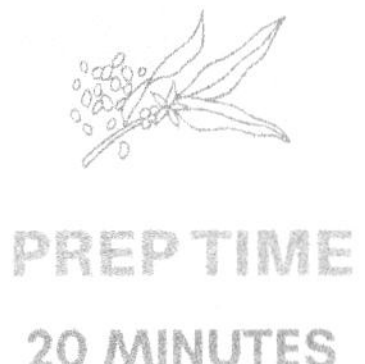

PREP TIME
20 MINUTES

COOK TIME
30 MINUTES

INGREDIENTS:

- 1 head green cabbage, shredded (about 4 cups)
- 1 carrot, peeled and grated (about 1 cup)
- 1/2 cup mayonnaise
- 2 tablespoons white vinegar
- 1 tablespoon white sugar
- 1 teaspoon salt
- 1/4 teaspoon black pepper

Coleslaw is a classic side dish that's easy for young chefs to make. It's a great way to introduce them to the concept of mixing a dressing with fresh vegetables. Serve the coleslaw alongside burgers, hot dogs, or as a topping for pulled pork sandwiches.

PROCEDURE:

1. In a large bowl, combine the shredded cabbage and grated carrot.

2. In a small bowl, whisk together the mayonnaise, white vinegar, sugar, salt, and black pepper.

3. Pour the dressing over the cabbage and carrot mixture and stir until everything is evenly coated.

4. Cover the bowl and refrigerate the coleslaw for at least 30 minutes, or up to 2 days, to allow the flavors to blend.

5. Stir the coleslaw again before serving.

Tips for young chefs:

- Let them help measure and add the ingredients.

- Demonstrate how to safely shred the cabbage and grate the carrot.

- Encourage them to taste the coleslaw and suggest adjustments to the dressing.

- Discuss the importance of food safety when handling raw vegetables.

45. CAESAR SALAD

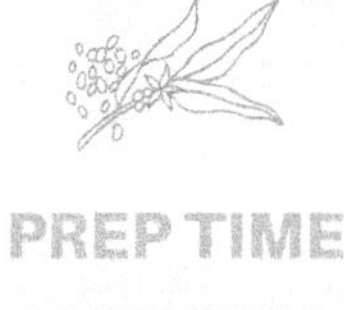

PREP TIME
20 MINUTES

COOK TIME
30 MINUTES

INGREDIENTS:

- 1 head romaine lettuce, washed and chopped
- 1/2 cup croutons
- 1/4 cup grated Parmesan cheese
- 2 tablespoons Caesar salad dressing
- 1 grilled or baked chicken breast, sliced (optional)

For the Dressing:
- 2 tablespoons mayonnaise
- 1 tablespoon lemon juice
- 1 teaspoon Dijon mustard
- 1 clove garlic, minced
- 1 tablespoon grated Parmesan cheese
- Salt and pepper to taste

PROCEDURE:

1. In a large bowl, combine the chopped romaine lettuce, croutons, and grated Parmesan cheese.

2. In a small bowl, whisk together the mayonnaise, lemon juice, Dijon mustard, minced garlic, and Parmesan cheese for the dressing. Season with salt and pepper to taste.

3. Drizzle the Caesar salad dressing over the lettuce mixture and toss gently to coat.

4. If using, top the salad with sliced grilled or baked chicken breast. Serve the Caesar salad immediately.

Tips for young chefs:

- Let them help wash and chop the romaine lettuce.

- Demonstrate how to safely use a grater to grate the Parmesan cheese.

- Encourage them to taste the dressing and suggest adjustments.

- Discuss the importance of food safety when handling raw ingredients.

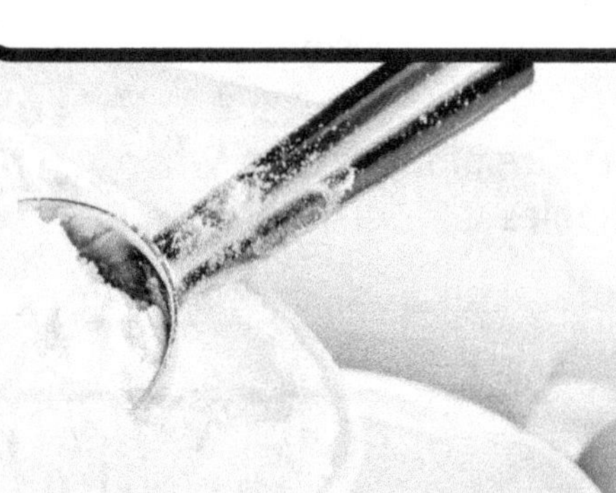

46. CORN ON THE COB

PREP TIME
20 MINUTES

COOK TIME
30 MINUTES

INGREDIENTS:

- 4•6 ears of fresh corn, husks and silk removed
- 2 tablespoons butter, softened
- Salt and pepper to taste

Tips for young chefs:

- Let them help remove the husks and silk from the corn.

- Demonstrate how to safely add the corn to the boiling water.

- Encourage them to taste the corn and suggest seasonings.

- Discuss the importance of food safety when handling hot items.

PROCEDURE:

1. Bring a large pot of water to a boil over high heat.

2. While the water is heating, use your hands to gently remove the husks and silk from the corn. Rinse the corn under cool water to remove any remaining silk.

3. Once the water is boiling, carefully add the corn cobs to the pot. Cover and cook for 5•7 minutes, or until the corn is tender.

4. Using tongs, carefully remove the cooked corn from the boiling water and place it on a serving platter.

5. Spread the softened butter evenly over the hot corn cobs.

6. Season the corn with salt and pepper to taste.

7. Serve the corn on the cob warm, with extra butter and seasonings on the side if desired.

Corn on the Cob is a classic, easy•to•prepare side dish that's perfect for young chefs. Encourage them to get creative by trying different seasoning blends or toppings, such as grated Parmesan cheese, chili powder, or fresh herbs.

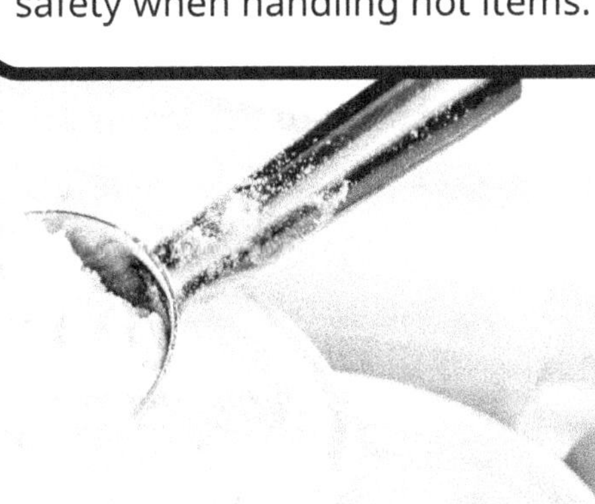

47. BAKED BEANS

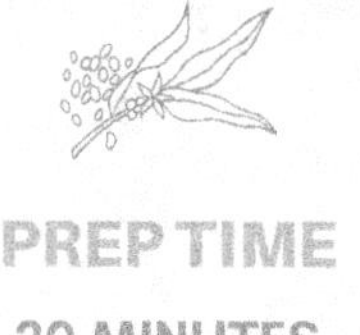

PREP TIME
20 MINUTES

COOK TIME
30 MINUTES

INGREDIENTS:

• 2 (15 oz) cans of navy or pinto beans, drained and rinsed
• 1/2 cup ketchup
• 2 tablespoons brown sugar
• 1 tablespoon Dijon mustard
• 1 teaspoon Worcestershire sauce
• 1/4 teaspoon garlic powder
• Salt and pepper to taste

Tips for young chefs:
• Let them help measure and add the ingredients to the bowl.

• Demonstrate how to properly drain and rinse the canned beans.

• Encourage them to taste the bean mixture and suggest seasonings.

• Discuss the importance of food safety when handling canned goods.

PROCEDURE:

1. Preheat your oven to 350°F (175°C).

2. In a large bowl, combine the drained and rinsed beans, ketchup, brown sugar, Dijon mustard, Worcestershire sauce, and garlic powder. Stir everything together until well mixed.

3. Transfer the bean mixture to a baking dish or casserole dish.

4. Bake the beans in the preheated oven for 30•40 minutes, or until the sauce has thickened and the beans are heated through.

5. Remove the baked beans from the oven and let them cool for a few minutes before serving.

6. Season the baked beans with salt and pepper to taste.

Baked Beans are a classic, kid•friendly side dish that's easy for young chefs to make. Serve the baked beans alongside hot dogs, burgers, or as part of a barbecue or picnic menu. You can also add cooked ground beef or bacon to the beans for extra flavor.

48. POTATO SALAD

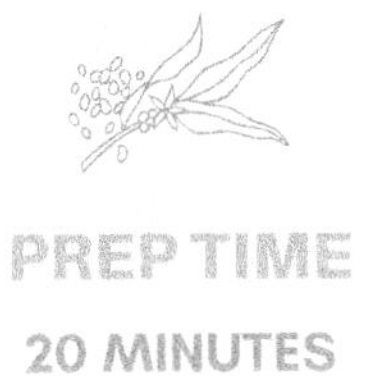

PREP TIME
20 MINUTES

COOK TIME
30 MINUTES

INGREDIENTS :

• 3 lbs Yukon Gold or red potatoes, peeled and cut into 1•inch cubes
• 1/2 cup mayonnaise
• 2 tablespoons Dijon mustard
• 2 tablespoons white vinegar
• 1/4 cup chopped onion
• 2 hard•boiled eggs, chopped
• 2 tablespoons chopped fresh parsley (optional)
• Salt and pepper to taste

Tips for young chefs:
• Let them help peel and cube the potatoes.

• Demonstrate how to safely boil and drain the potatoes.

• Encourage them to taste the dressing and suggest seasonings.

• Discuss the importance of food safety when handling raw ingredients

PROCEDURE :

1. Place the cubed potatoes in a large pot and cover with cold water. Bring the water to a boil over high heat.

2. Reduce the heat to medium•low and simmer the potatoes for 10•15 minutes, or until they are tender when pierced with a fork. Drain the potatoes and let them cool completely.

3. In a large bowl, whisk together the mayonnaise, Dijon mustard, and white vinegar until well combined.

4. Add the cooled, cooked potatoes, chopped onion, chopped hard•boiled eggs, and parsley (if using) to the dressing. Gently toss everything together until the potatoes are evenly coated.

5. Season the potato salad with salt and pepper to taste.

6. Cover the bowl and refrigerate the potato salad for at least 30 minutes, or up to 2 days, to allow the flavors to blend.

7. Serve the potato salad chilled or at room temperature.

49. GREEN BEAN ALMONDINE

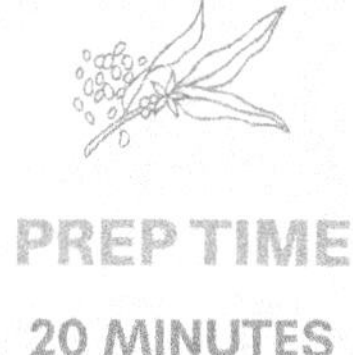

PREP TIME
20 MINUTES

COOK TIME
30 MINUTES

INGREDIENTS:

- 1 lb fresh green beans, trimmed
- 2 tablespoons butter
- 1/4 cup sliced almonds
- 1 clove garlic, minced
- 1 tablespoon lemon juice
- Salt and pepper to taste

Tips for young chefs:

- Let them help trim the green beans and measure the ingredients.

- Demonstrate how to safely use a knife to mince the garlic.

- Encourage them to taste the dish and suggest seasonings.

- Discuss the importance of food safety when handling hot items.

PROCEDURE:

1. Bring a large pot of salted water to a boil. Add the trimmed green beans and cook for 5•7 minutes, until tender•crisp. Drain the beans and set them aside.

2. In a skillet, melt the butter over medium heat. Add the sliced almonds and minced garlic. Cook, stirring frequently, for 2•3 minutes, until the almonds are lightly toasted and the garlic is fragrant.

3. Add the cooked green beans to the skillet with the toasted almonds and garlic. Drizzle the lemon juice over the top and toss everything together gently to coat the beans.

4. Season the Green Bean Almondine with salt and pepper to taste.

5. Serve the Green Bean Almondine warm.

Green Bean Almondine is a simple, flavorful side dish that's easy for young chefs to prepare. The toasted almonds and lemon juice add a delicious crunch and brightness to the tender green beans. Serve this dish alongside roasted meats, fish, or as part of a larger meal.

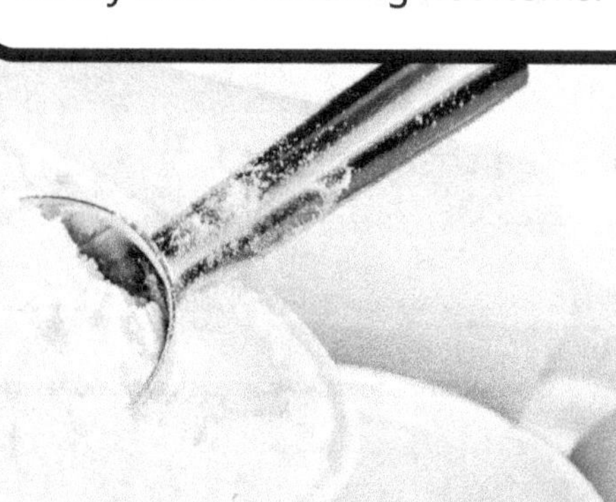

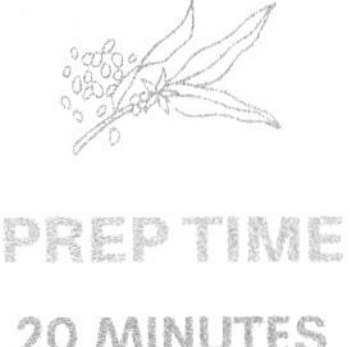

50. BRUSSELS SPROUTS WITH BACON

PREP TIME
20 MINUTES

COOK TIME
30 MINUTES

INGREDIENTS:

• 1 lb Brussels sprouts, trimmed and halved
• 4 slices of bacon, chopped
• 1 tablespoon olive oil
• 1 clove garlic, minced
• Salt and pepper to taste

Tips for young chefs:
• Let them help trim and halve the Brussels sprouts.

• Demonstrate how to safely cook the bacon and add the other ingredients.

• Encourage them to taste the dish and suggest seasonings.

• Discuss the importance of food safety when handling hot items.

PROCEDURE:

1. In a large skillet, cook the chopped bacon over medium heat until crispy, about 5•7 minutes. Transfer the cooked bacon to a paper towel•lined plate, leaving the bacon grease in the skillet.

2. Add the olive oil to the skillet with the bacon grease. Increase the heat to medium•high and add the halved Brussels sprouts. Cook, stirring occasionally, for 5•7 minutes, until the Brussels sprouts are starting to brown.

3. Reduce the heat to medium, add the minced garlic, and continue cooking for 2•3 minutes, until the garlic is fragrant.

4. Add the cooked bacon back to the skillet and toss everything together until well combined.

5. Season the Brussels sprouts with salt and pepper to taste.

6. Serve the Brussels Sprouts with Bacon hot.

Brussels Sprouts with Bacon is a simple, flavorful side dish that's easy for young chefs to prepare. The crispy bacon adds a delicious savory element to the tender Brussels sprouts. Serve this dish alongside roasted meats, pasta, or as part of a larger meal.

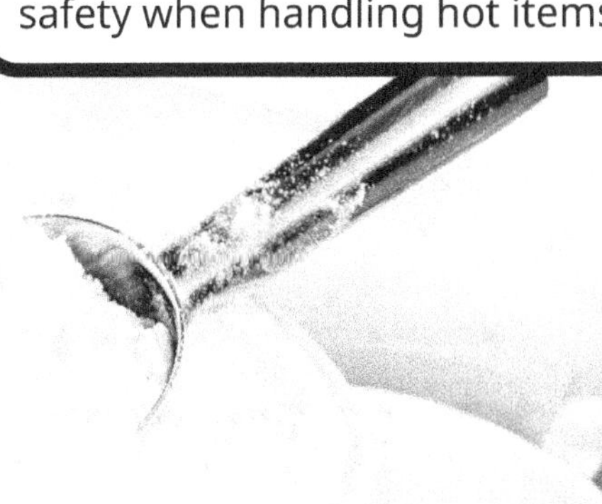

51. CHOCOLATE CHIP COOKIES

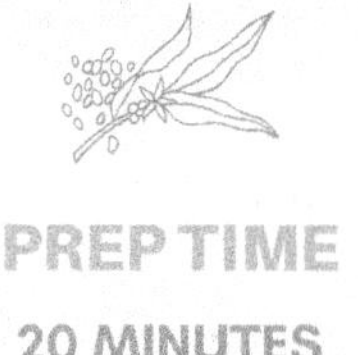

PREP TIME

20 MINUTES

COOK TIME

30 MINUTES

INGREDIENTS :

- 2 1/4 cups all•purpose flour
- 1 teaspoon baking soda
- 1 teaspoon salt
- 1 cup (2 sticks) unsalted butter, softened
- 3/4 cup granulated sugar
- 3/4 cup packed brown sugar
- 1 teaspoon vanilla extract
- 2 large eggs
- 2 cups semi•sweet chocolate chips

Tips for young chefs:

- Let them help measure and add the ingredients.
- Demonstrate how to properly cream the butter and sugars.
- Encourage them to taste the dough and suggest mix•ins.
- Discuss the importance of food safety when handling raw eggs.

PROCEDURE :

1. Preheat your oven to 375°F (190°C). Line baking sheets with parchment paper.

2. In a medium bowl, whisk together the flour, baking soda, and salt. Set aside.

3. In a large bowl, beat the softened butter, granulated sugar, and brown sugar together until light and fluffy, about 2•3 minutes.

4. Beat in the vanilla extract and then the eggs, one at a time, until well combined.

5. Gradually stir the dry ingredients into the wet ingredients until just combined. Fold in the chocolate chips.

6. Scoop rounded tablespoons of dough onto the prepared baking sheets, spacing them about 2 inches apart.

7. Bake the cookies for 10•12 minutes, or until the edges are lightly golden brown.

8. Allow the cookies to cool on the baking sheets for 5 minutes before transferring them to a wire rack to cool completely.

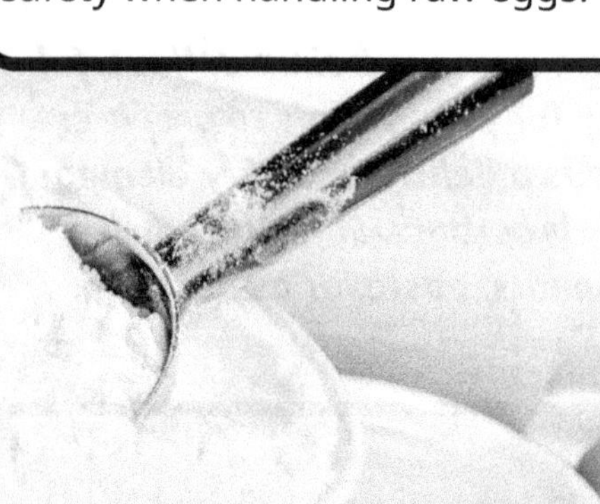

52. BROWNIES

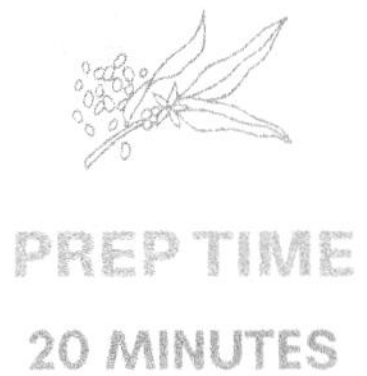

INGREDIENTS :

- 1/2 cup (1 stick) unsalted butter, melted
- 1 cup granulated sugar
- 2 large eggs
- 1 teaspoon vanilla extract
- 1/3 cup all•purpose flour
- 1/4 cup unsweetened cocoa powder
- 1/4 teaspoon salt
- 1/2 cup semi•sweet chocolate chips (optional)

Tips for young chefs:

- Let them help measure and add the ingredients.
- Demonstrate how to properly melt the butter and whisk the batter.
- Encourage them to taste the batter and suggest mix•ins.
- Discuss the importance of food safety when handling raw eggs.

PROCEDURE :

1. Preheat your oven to 350°F (175°C). Grease an 8x8•inch baking pan with butter or non•stick cooking spray.

2. In a medium bowl, whisk together the melted butter and granulated sugar until well combined.

3. Beat in the eggs, one at a time, then stir in the vanilla extract.

4. In a separate bowl, whisk together the flour, cocoa powder, and salt.

5. Gradually stir the dry ingredients into the wet ingredients until just combined. Do not overmix.

6. If using, fold in the chocolate chips.

7. Spread the brownie batter evenly into the prepared baking pan.

8. Bake the brownies for 25•30 minutes, or until a toothpick inserted into the center comes out with a few moist crumbs.

9. Allow the brownies to cool completely in the pan before cutting into squares.

53. CUPCAKES

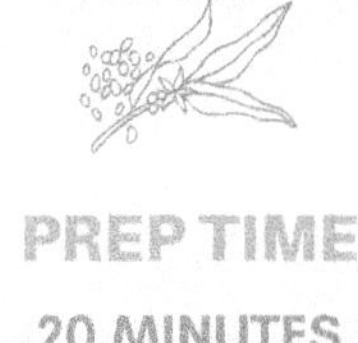

PREP TIME
20 MINUTES

COOK TIME
30 MINUTES

INGREDIENTS:

• 4•6 ears of fresh corn, husks and silk removed
• 2 tablespoons butter, softened
• Salt and pepper to taste

Tips for young chefs:

• Let them help measure and add the ingredients.

• Demonstrate how to properly cream the butter and sugar.

• Encourage them to taste the batter and suggest mix•ins.

• Discuss the importance of food safety when handling raw eggs.

PROCEDURE:

1. Preheat your oven to 350°F (175°C). Line a 12•cup muffin tin with paper liners. In a medium bowl, whisk together the flour, baking powder, and salt. Set aside.

2. In a large bowl, beat the softened butter and granulated sugar together until light and fluffy, about 2•3 minutes. Beat in the eggs, one at a time, then stir in the vanilla extract.

3. Alternate adding the flour mixture and milk to the butter mixture, mixing just until combined after each addition. Divide the batter evenly among the prepared muffin cups, filling them about 3/4 full.

4. Bake the cupcakes for 18•20 minutes, or until a toothpick inserted into the center comes out clean.

5. Allow the cupcakes to cool in the muffin tin for 5 minutes, then transfer them to a wire rack to cool completely.

6. For the frosting, beat the softened butter in a large bowl until smooth. Gradually add the confectioners' sugar, 1•2 tablespoons of milk, and the vanilla extract, beating until the frosting is light and fluffy. Frost the cooled cupcakes and serve.

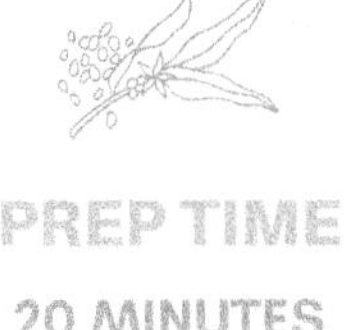

54. RICE KRISPIE TREATS

PREP TIME
20 MINUTES

COOK TIME
30 MINUTES

INGREDIENTS:

- 3 tablespoons unsalted butter
- 4 cups miniature marshmallows
- 6 cups Rice Krispies cereal
- Pinch of salt (optional)

Tips for young chefs:
- Let them help measure and add the ingredients.

- Demonstrate how to safely melt the butter and marshmallows.

- Encourage them to be creative with mix•ins, like chocolate chips or sprinkles.

- Discuss the importance of food safety when handling hot items.

PROCEDURE:

1. Grease an 8x8•inch baking pan with butter or non•stick cooking spray.

2. In a large saucepan, melt the 3 tablespoons of butter over medium heat.

3. Once the butter is melted, add the marshmallows and stir constantly until they are completely melted and the mixture is smooth.

4. Remove the saucepan from the heat and immediately add the Rice Krispies cereal. Stir quickly to coat the cereal evenly with the marshmallow mixture.

5. Using a greased spatula or your hands, press the Rice Krispie mixture into the prepared baking pan, smoothing the top. If desired, sprinkle a pinch of salt over the top.

6. Allow the Rice Krispie Treats to cool completely, about 30 minutes, before cutting into squares. Serve the Rice Krispie Treats and enjoy!

Rice Krispie Treats are a classic, no•bake dessert that's perfect for young chefs. The simple ingredients and hands•on assembly make it a great recipe for kids to get involved in. Encourage them to experiment with different flavors and toppings to make their own unique treats.

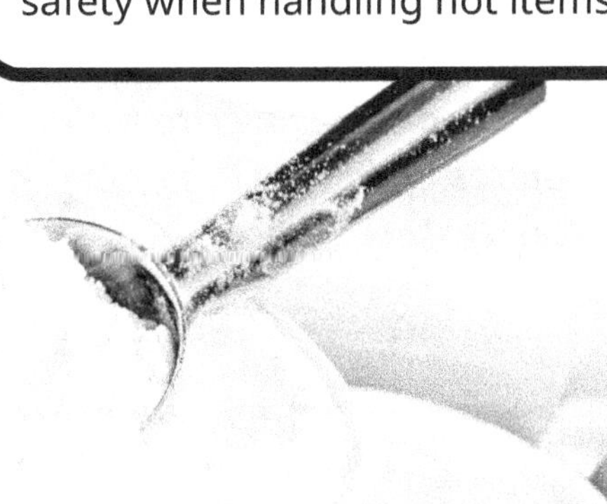

55. FRUIT POPSICLES

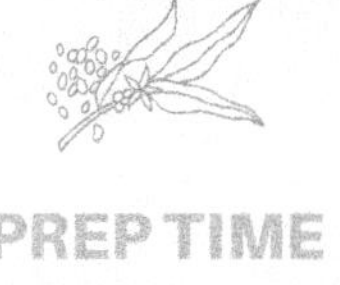 

PREP TIME
20 MINUTES

COOK TIME
30 MINUTES

INGREDIENTS:

• 2 cups chopped fresh fruit (such as strawberries, blueberries, mango, or pineapple)
• 1/2 cup 100% fruit juice (such as orange, apple, or grape juice)
• 2 tablespoons honey (optional)

Tips for young chefs:

• Let them help choose and chop the fresh fruit.

• Demonstrate how to safely use a blender to puree the fruit.

• Encourage them to experiment with different fruit and juice combinations.

• Discuss the importance of food safety when handling frozen items.

PROCEDURE:

1. In a blender, puree the chopped fruit and fruit juice until smooth. Taste and add honey if desired, blending again to incorporate.

2. Carefully pour the fruit mixture into popsicle molds, leaving a small amount of space at the top for expansion.

3. Insert popsicle sticks into the molds, making sure they are centered and secure.

4. Freeze the popsicles for at least 4 hours, or until completely frozen.

5. To remove the popsicles from the molds, run the molds under warm water for 30 seconds to 1 minute, then gently pull the popsicles out.

6. Serve the Fruit Popsicles immediately or store them in an airtight container in the freezer for up to 2 months.

Fruit Popsicles are a refreshing, healthy treat that's easy for young chefs to make. Encourage them to get creative by using their favorite fruits or even adding small pieces of fruit to the popsicle molds for a fun, textured treat.

56. CHOCOLATE PUDDING

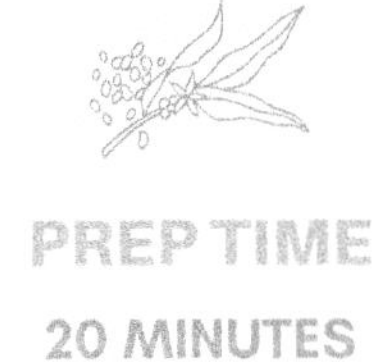

PREP TIME
20 MINUTES

COOK TIME
30 MINUTES

INGREDIENTS:

- 2 cups whole milk
- 1/4 cup granulated sugar
- 2 tablespoons unsweetened cocoa powder
- 2 tablespoons cornstarch
- 1/4 teaspoon salt
- 2 ounces semisweet chocolate, chopped
- 1 teaspoon vanilla extract

Tips for young chefs:

- Let them help measure and add the ingredients.
- Demonstrate how to properly whisk the pudding mixture as it cooks.
- Encourage them to taste the pudding and suggest additional flavorings.
- Discuss the importance of food safety when handling hot items.

PROCEDURE:

1. In a medium saucepan, whisk together the milk, sugar, cocoa powder, cornstarch, and salt.

2. Place the saucepan over medium heat and cook, whisking constantly, until the mixture thickens and comes to a boil, about 5•7 minutes.

3. Remove the saucepan from the heat and stir in the chopped semisweet chocolate until it's melted and the pudding is smooth.

4. Stir in the vanilla extract. Divide the hot chocolate pudding into individual serving dishes or ramekins.

6. Cover the surface of the pudding with plastic wrap to prevent a skin from forming.

7. Refrigerate the pudding for at least 2 hours, or until it's completely chilled and set.

8. Serve the chocolate pudding cold, with whipped cream or a sprinkle of cocoa powder on top, if desired.

Chocolate Pudding is a classic, creamy dessert that's easy for young chefs to make. Encourage them to get creative by adding their favorite mix•ins, such as crushed cookies, chopped nuts, or a drizzle of caramel sauce.

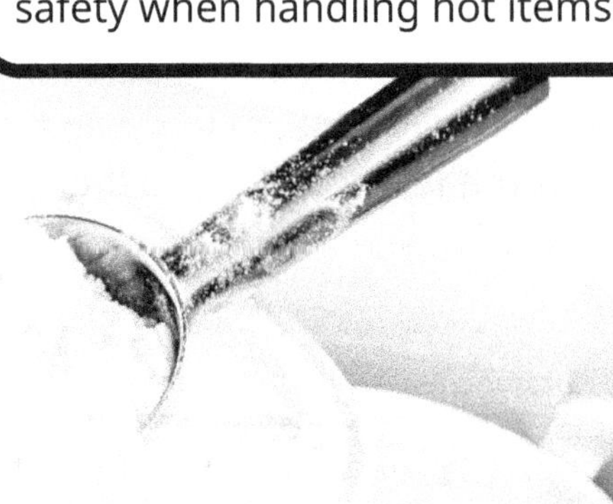

57. APPLE PIE

<table>
<tr><td>PREP TIME</td><td>COOK TIME</td></tr>
<tr><td>20 MINUTES</td><td>30 MINUTES</td></tr>
</table>

INGREDIENTS:

Pie Crust:
- 2 1/2 cups all•purpose flour
- 1 teaspoon salt
- 3/4 cup (1 1/2 sticks) unsalted butter, chilled and cubed
- 1/4 cup ice water

Filling:
- 6 cups peeled, cored, and sliced Granny Smith apples (about 6•8 apples)
- 3/4 cup granulated sugar
- 2 tablespoons all•purpose flour
- 1 teaspoon ground cinnamon
- 1/4 teaspoon ground nutmeg
- 1 tablespoon unsalted butter, cubed

7. Bake the pie for 20 minutes, then reduce the oven temperature to 350°F (175°C) and bake for an additional 30•40 minutes, or until the crust is golden brown and the filling is bubbly.

8. Allow the pie to cool completely before slicing and serving.

PROCEDURE:

1. Make the pie crust: In a food processor, pulse the flour and salt together. Add the chilled butter cubes and pulse until the mixture resembles coarse crumbs. Slowly add the ice water and pulse just until the dough begins to come together. Divide the dough in half, shape each half into a disk, wrap in plastic, and refrigerate for at least 1 hour.

2. Preheat your oven to 400°F (200°C).

3. Make the filling: In a large bowl, toss the sliced apples with the sugar, flour, cinnamon, and nutmeg until well coated.

4. On a lightly floured surface, roll out one disk of dough into a 12•inch circle. Carefully transfer the dough to a 9•inch pie plate. Trim the excess dough, leaving about 1 inch of overhang.

5. Spoon the apple filling into the pie crust and dot the top with the cubed butter.

6. Roll out the remaining dough disk into a 12•inch circle. Cut slits in the top to allow steam to escape. Place the top crust over the filling and crimp the edges to seal.

58. BANANA SPLIT

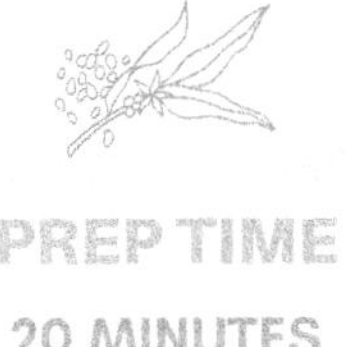

PREP TIME
20 MINUTES

COOK TIME
30 MINUTES

INGREDIENTS:

• 2 ripe bananas, peeled and cut in half lengthwise
• 2 scoops vanilla ice cream
• 2 scoops chocolate ice cream
• 2 scoops strawberry ice cream
• Whipped cream
• Chocolate syrup
• Maraschino cherries
• Chopped nuts (optional)

Tips for young chefs:
• Let them help peel and cut the bananas.

• Demonstrate how to scoop the ice cream neatly.

• Encourage them to be creative with the toppings and placement.

• Discuss the importance of food safety when handling cold items.

PROCEDURE:

1. Place the banana halves in a long dish or on a plate.

2. Scoop the vanilla, chocolate, and strawberry ice cream onto the banana halves, arranging them in a row.

3. Top the ice cream with a generous dollop of whipped cream.

4. Drizzle the chocolate syrup over the whipped cream and ice cream.

5. Top each banana split with a maraschino cherry.

6. If desired, sprinkle chopped nuts over the top.

7. Serve the banana split immediately, with extra toppings on the side.

The Banana Split is a classic, fun dessert that's perfect for young chefs to make. Encourage them to get involved in the assembly process and let them customize their creations with their favorite toppings. This recipe is a great way to get kids excited about making their own desserts.

59. ICE CREAM SUNDAES

PREP TIME
20 MINUTES

COOK TIME
30 MINUTES

INGREDIENTS :

- Vanilla ice cream
- Chocolate syrup
- Whipped cream
- Maraschino cherries
- Sprinkles or crushed cookies (optional)

Ice Cream Sundaes are a classic, fun dessert that's perfect for young chefs to make. Encourage them to get creative by offering a variety of toppings, such as crushed nuts, caramel sauce, or chopped fruit. This is a great way to let kids' imaginations run wild and customize their own sweet treat.

PROCEDURE :

1. Scoop 1•2 scoops of vanilla ice cream into a bowl or sundae dish.

2. Drizzle the chocolate syrup over the ice cream.

3. Top the ice cream with a dollop of whipped cream.

4. Place a maraschino cherry on top of the whipped cream.

5. If desired, sprinkle some colorful sprinkles or crushed cookies over the sundae.

6. Serve the Ice Cream Sundae immediately, with any extra toppings on the side.

Tips for young chefs:
- Let them help scoop the ice cream and add the toppings.

- Demonstrate how to properly use a spoon to drizzle the chocolate syrup.

- Encourage them to be creative with the toppings and placement.

- Discuss the importance of food safety when handling cold items.

60. PEACH COBBLER

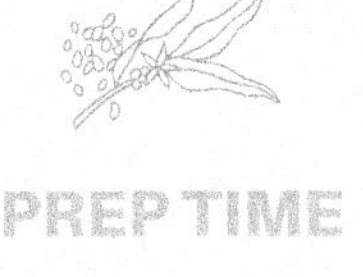

PREP TIME
20 MINUTES

COOK TIME
30 MINUTES

INGREDIENTS:

• 4 cups sliced fresh peaches (or 2 (15 oz) cans of peach slices, drained)
• 1/2 cup granulated sugar
• 1 tablespoon all•purpose flour
• 1/2 teaspoon ground cinnamon
• 1/4 teaspoon ground nutmeg

Topping:
• 1 cup all•purpose flour
• 1/4 cup granulated sugar
• 2 teaspoons baking powder
• 1/4 teaspoon salt
• 4 tablespoons unsalted butter, chilled and cubed
• 1/2 cup milk

Tips for young chefs:
• Let them help measure and mix the ingredients.

• Demonstrate how to safely use a pastry blender or forks to cut in the butter.

PROCEDURE:

1. Preheat your oven to 375°F (190°C).

2. In a large bowl, gently toss the sliced peaches with the 1/2 cup of sugar, 1 tablespoon of flour, cinnamon, and nutmeg until well combined.

3. Transfer the peach mixture to a 9•inch baking dish.

4. In a medium bowl, whisk together the 1 cup of flour, 1/4 cup of sugar, baking powder, and salt.

5. Cut in the chilled, cubed butter using a pastry blender or two forks until the mixture resembles coarse crumbs.

6. Stir in the 1/2 cup of milk just until a soft dough forms.

7. Drop the dough by large spoonfuls onto the peach mixture, covering the top as much as possible.

8. Bake the Peach Cobbler for 30•35 minutes, or until the topping is golden brown and the peach filling is bubbly.

9. Allow the cobbler to cool for 10•15 minutes before serving.

61. LEMONADE

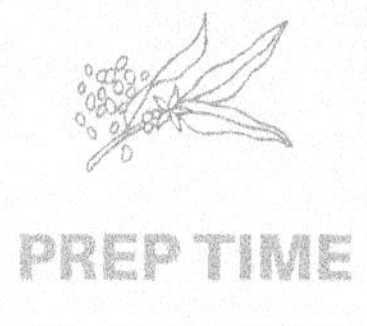

PREP TIME
20 MINUTES

COOK TIME
30 MINUTES

INGREDIENTS:

• 6 lemons, juiced (about 1 cup of lemon juice)
• 1/2 cup sugar
• 4 cups cold water
• Ice cubes
• Lemon slices for garnish (optional)

PROCEDURE:

1. In a pitcher, stir together the lemon juice and sugar until the sugar is fully dissolved.

2. Add the 4 cups of cold water and stir to combine.

3. Taste the lemonade and add more sugar if it's too tart, or more water if it's too sweet.

4. Fill glasses with ice cubes and pour the lemonade over the ice.

5. Garnish with lemon slices, if desired.

Tips for Young Chefs:

• Let them measure and add the ingredients themselves.

• Encourage them to experiment with the lemon•to•sugar ratio to find their perfect balance of sweet and tart.

• Suggest they get creative by adding fresh mint, sliced strawberries, or a splash of club soda.

• Provide supervision when juicing the lemons, as the juice can squirt.

62. ICED TEA

PREP TIME
20 MINUTES

COOK TIME
30 MINUTES

INGREDIENTS:

- 4 tea bags (black, green, or herbal tea)
- 4 cups water
- 2•3 tablespoons sugar (or to taste)
- Lemon slices (optional)
- Ice cubes

Tips for Young Chefs:

- Let them measure and add the ingredients themselves.

- Encourage them to experiment with different types of tea.

- Suggest they get creative by adding fresh mint, sliced fruit, or a splash of lemon or lime juice.

- Provide supervision when using the stove.

PROCEDURE:

1. In a medium saucepan, bring the 4 cups of water to a boil.

2. Once the water is boiling, remove the pan from the heat and add the 4 tea bags.

3. Let the tea steep for 5•7 minutes, then remove the tea bags.

4. Stir in the 2•3 tablespoons of sugar until it's fully dissolved.

5. Pour the sweetened tea into a pitcher and refrigerate until completely chilled, about 2•3 hours.

6. Fill glasses with ice cubes and pour the chilled tea over the ice.

7. Garnish with lemon slices, if desired.

Enjoy your refreshing homemade iced tea!

63. SMOOTHIES

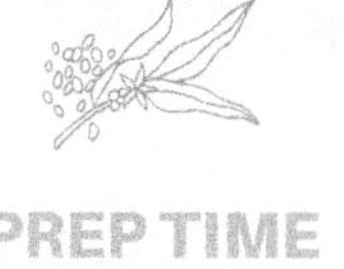 

PREP TIME
20 MINUTES

COOK TIME
30 MINUTES

INGREDIENTS:

- 1 cup milk or non•dairy milk (such as almond or oat milk)
- 1 cup frozen fruit (such as strawberries, blueberries, or banana)
- 1/2 cup plain yogurt
- 1 tablespoon honey (optional)

PROCEDURE:

1. Add the milk, frozen fruit, and yogurt to a blender.

2. If desired, add the honey and blend until smooth and creamy.

3. Pour the smoothie into glasses and serve immediately.

Tips for young chefs:

- Let them help measure and add the ingredients to the blender.

- Demonstrate how to safely use the blender.

- Encourage them to experiment with different fruit and milk combinations.

- Discuss the importance of food safety when handling blenders.

Smoothies are a fun, healthy, and easy•to•make treat that's perfect for young chefs. Encourage them to get creative by adding their favorite fruits, vegetables, or even a spoonful of peanut butter or cocoa powder. Smoothies are a great way to get kids to enjoy a nutritious snack or breakfast.

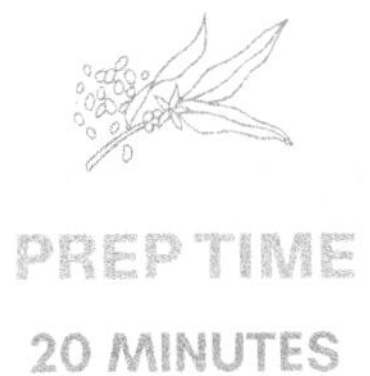

64. MILKSHAKES

PREP TIME
20 MINUTES

COOK TIME
30 MINUTES

INGREDIENTS:

- 2 cups cold milk (dairy, almond, or oat milk)
- 2 scoops ice cream (vanilla, chocolate, or strawberry)
- 1/2 teaspoon vanilla extract (optional)
- Whipped cream (optional)
- Cherries, sprinkles, or other toppings (optional)

PROCEDURE:

1. Add the milk, ice cream, and vanilla extract (if using) to a blender.

2. Blend on high speed until the mixture is smooth and creamy, about 30 seconds to 1 minute.

3. Pour the milkshake into a tall glass.

4. Top with whipped cream and any other desired toppings, such as cherries, sprinkles, or chocolate syrup.

Tips for Young Chefs:

- Let them measure and add the ingredients themselves.

- Encourage them to experiment with different flavors of ice cream.

- Suggest they get creative by adding a spoonful of peanut butter, a banana, or a few drops of food coloring.

- Provide supervision when using the blender.

Enjoy your homemade milkshake!

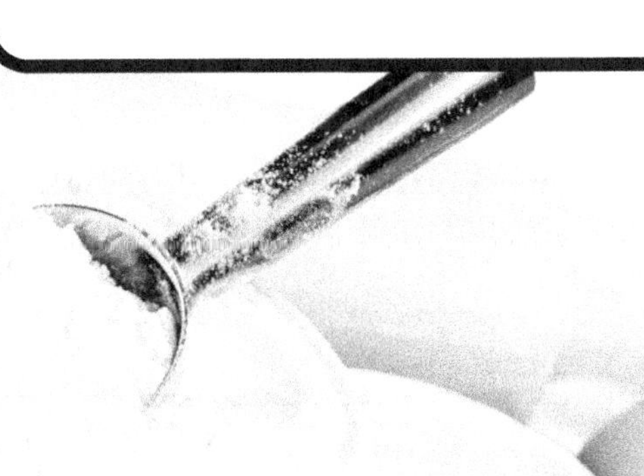

65. HOT CHOCOLATE

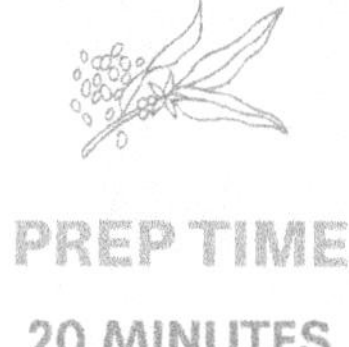 

INGREDIENTS:

- 2 cups milk (dairy, almond, or oat milk)
- 2 tablespoons unsweetened cocoa powder
- 2 tablespoons sugar (or to taste)
- 1/4 teaspoon vanilla extract (optional)
- Whipped cream (optional)
- Marshmallows (optional)

PROCEDURE:

1. In a small saucepan, whisk together the milk, cocoa powder, and sugar.

2. Heat the mixture over medium heat, stirring frequently, until it starts to steam and bubble slightly around the edges. Do not let it boil.

3. Remove the saucepan from the heat and stir in the vanilla extract, if using.

4. Carefully pour the hot chocolate into mugs.

5. Top with whipped cream and/or marshmallows, if desired.

Tips for Young Chefs:

- Let them measure and add the ingredients themselves.

- Encourage them to taste the hot chocolate and add more sugar if needed.

- Provide supervision when using the stove.

- Suggest they get creative by adding a sprinkle of cinnamon, a dash of peppermint extract, or a few chocolate chips on top.

66. FRUIT PUNCH

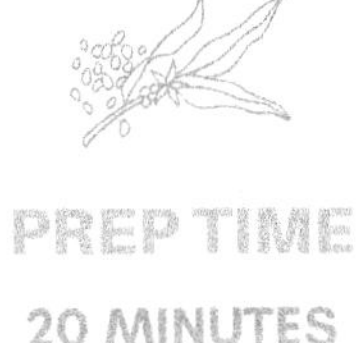

PREP TIME
20 MINUTES

COOK TIME
30 MINUTES

INGREDIENTS:

- 2 cups pineapple juice
- 2 cups orange juice
- 1 cup cranberry juice
- 1 cup grape juice
- 1 cup cold water
- 1 liter of lemon•lime soda (such as Sprite or 7•Up)
- Ice cubes
- Fruit slices for garnish (optional)

PROCEDURE:

1. In a large pitcher, combine the pineapple juice, orange juice, cranberry juice, grape juice, and cold water. Stir well to mix.

2. Just before serving, add the lemon•lime soda and stir gently to combine.

3. Fill glasses with ice cubes.

4. Ladle or pour the fruit punch over the ice.

5. Garnish with slices of fruit, such as orange, lemon, or pineapple, if desired.

Tips for Young Chefs:

• Let them measure and add the ingredients themselves.

• Encourage them to experiment with different juice combinations to find their favorite flavor.

• Suggest they get creative by adding a splash of grenadine for a pink hue or frozen fruit instead of ice cubes.

• Provide supervision when handling the glass pitcher and pouring the punch.

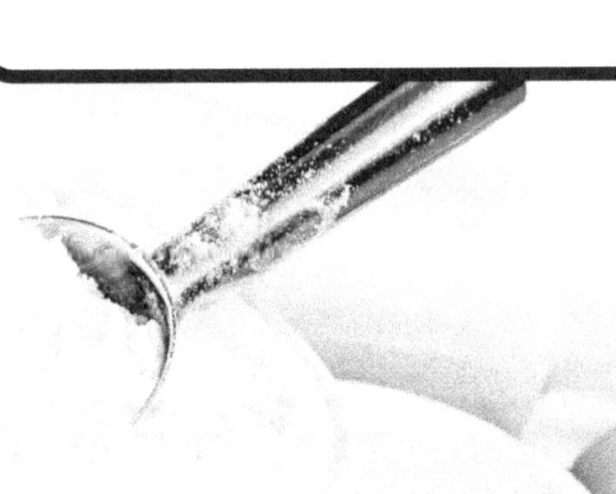

67. MANGO LASSI

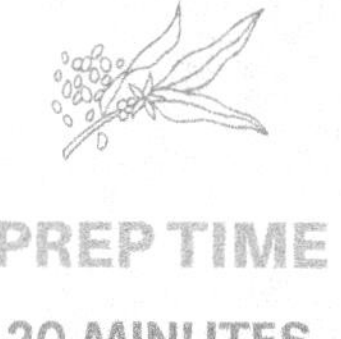

PREP TIME
20 MINUTES

COOK TIME
30 MINUTES

INGREDIENTS :

• 1 ripe mango, peeled and diced (about 1 cup)
• 1 cup plain yogurt
• 1/2 cup milk
• 2•3 tablespoons sugar (or to taste)
• 1/4 teaspoon ground cardamom (optional)
• Ice cubes (optional)

PROCEDURE :

1. In a blender, combine the diced mango, yogurt, milk, and sugar. Blend until smooth and creamy.

2. If using, add the ground cardamom and blend again briefly to incorporate.

3. Taste the lassi and add more sugar if needed, blending again to combine.

4. Pour the mango lassi into glasses.

5. If desired, add a few ice cubes to each glass.

Tips for Young Chefs:

• Let them measure and add the ingredients themselves.

• Encourage them to taste the lassi and adjust the sweetness to their liking.

• Suggest they get creative by adding a sprinkle of cinnamon or a few mint leaves as a garnish.

• Provide supervision when using the blender.

68. ARNOLD PALMER (LEMONADE AND ICED TEA)

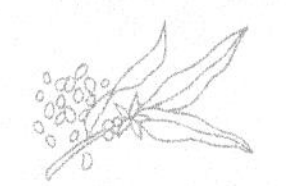

PREP TIME
20 MINUTES

COOK TIME
30 MINUTES

INGREDIENTS:

- 1 cup freshly brewed black tea, cooled
- 1 cup lemonade
- Ice cubes

PROCEDURE:

1. In a pitcher or large glass, combine the brewed black tea and lemonade.

2. Stir the mixture gently to combine.

3. Fill glasses with ice cubes. Pour the Arnold Palmer over the ice and serve immediately.

Tips for young chefs:

• Let them help measure and combine the tea and lemonade.

• Demonstrate how to properly brew the black tea and let it cool.

• Encourage them to taste the drink and suggest adjustments to the ratio of tea to lemonade.

• Discuss the importance of food safety when handling hot liquids.

The Arnold Palmer is a refreshing, classic non•alcoholic drink that's easy for young chefs to make. Encourage them to experiment with different types of tea or lemonade to find their perfect flavor combination. This drink is perfect for warm weather or as a accompaniment to a meal.

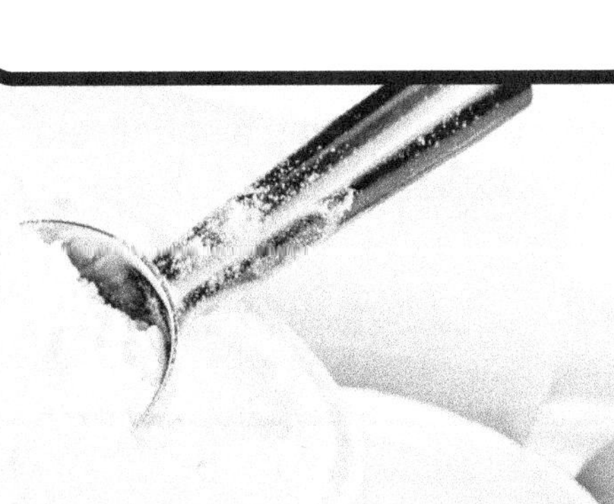

69. WATERMELON JUICE

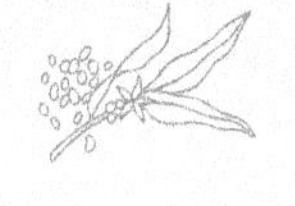

PREP TIME
20 MINUTES

COOK TIME
30 MINUTES

INGREDIENTS:

- 4 cups cubed watermelon (about 1/2 a small watermelon)
- 1•2 tablespoons sugar (optional, to taste)
- Ice cubes (optional)

PROCEDURE:

1. In a blender, add the cubed watermelon.

2. Blend on high speed until the watermelon is completely pureed and smooth, about 1 minute.

3. Taste the watermelon juice and add 1•2 tablespoons of sugar if desired, blending again briefly to incorporate.

4. Pour the watermelon juice through a fine mesh strainer to remove any foam or pulp, if desired.

5. Fill glasses with ice cubes, if using.

6. Carefully pour the strained watermelon juice over the ice.

Tips for Young Chefs:
- Let them measure and add the ingredients themselves.

- Encourage them to taste the juice and decide if they want to add any sugar.

- Suggest they get creative by adding a squeeze of lime juice or a few mint leaves as a garnish.

- Provide supervision when using the blender.

70. HOMEMADE HOT APPLE CIDER

INGREDIENTS:

- 4 cups apple juice or cider
- 1 cinnamon stick
- 3 whole cloves
- 1 orange, sliced
- 2 tablespoons honey (optional)

PROCEDURE:

1. In a medium saucepan, combine the apple juice or cider, cinnamon stick, whole cloves, and orange slices.

2. Heat the mixture over medium heat, stirring occasionally, until it starts to steam and bubble slightly around the edges. Do not let it boil.

3. Reduce the heat to low and let the cider simmer for 10•15 minutes, allowing the flavors to infuse.

4. Carefully remove the cinnamon stick and cloves.

5. If desired, stir in 2 tablespoons of honey to sweeten the cider.

6. Ladle the hot apple cider into mugs.

7. Garnish each mug with an orange slice, if desired.

Tips for Young Chefs:
- Let them measure and add the ingredients themselves.
- Encourage them to smell the cinnamon and cloves as the cider simmers.
- Suggest they get creative by adding a splash of brandy or rum for an adult version.
- Provide supervision when using the stove.

71. HAM AND CHEESE SANDWICHES

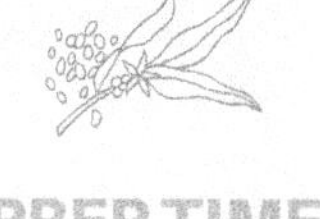 

PREP TIME
20 MINUTES

COOK TIME
30 MINUTES

INGREDIENTS :

- 4 slices of bread (white, wheat, or sourdough)
- 2 slices of ham
- 2 slices of cheese (cheddar, Swiss, or American)
- Butter or margarine (optional)

PROCEDURE :

1. Lay the 4 slices of bread out on a clean, flat surface.

2. Place 1 slice of ham on 2 of the bread slices.

3. Place 1 slice of cheese on top of the ham on each of those 2 slices.

4. Close the sandwiches by placing the remaining 2 bread slices on top.

5. If desired, spread a small amount of butter or margarine on the outside of the bread slices.

6. Heat a skillet or griddle over medium heat. Place the sandwiches in the hot pan and cook for 2•3 minutes per side, or until the bread is golden brown and the cheese is melted.

7. Carefully remove the sandwiches from the pan and let cool for a minute before serving.

Tips:
- Let young chefs customize their sandwiches by choosing their favorite types of ham and cheese.
- Encourage them to experiment with different bread types as well.
- Provide supervision when using the hot pan.

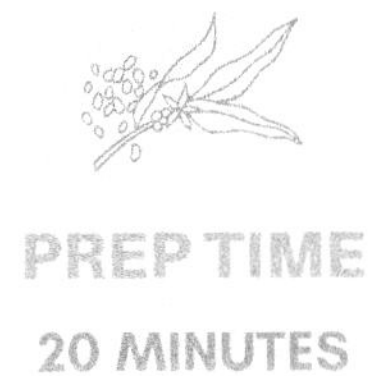

72. BLTS

PREP TIME
20 MINUTES

COOK TIME
30 MINUTES

INGREDIENTS:

• 8 slices of bread (white, wheat, or sourdough)
• 8 slices of cooked bacon
• 2 tomatoes, sliced
• 4 leaves of lettuce, washed and dried
• 2 tbsp mayonnaise
• Salt and pepper to taste

PROCEDURE:

1. Cook the bacon in a skillet or on a baking sheet until crispy. Drain on paper towels.

2. Lay 4 slices of bread on a clean surface.

3. Spread 1 tbsp of mayonnaise on each of the 4 bread slices.

4. Layer 2 slices of bacon, 2•3 tomato slices, and 1 lettuce leaf on each of the 4 bread slices.

5. Top each sandwich with another slice of bread.

6. Repeat the layering process with the remaining ingredients to create 4 complete BLT sandwiches.

Tips for Young Chefs:

• Let them measure and assemble the sandwiches themselves.

• Encourage them to experiment with different types of bread or add•ins like avocado or cheese.

• Suggest they get creative by adding a drizzle of balsamic glaze or a sprinkle of fresh herbs.

• Provide supervision when cooking the bacon and handling the sharp knife for slicing the tomatoes.

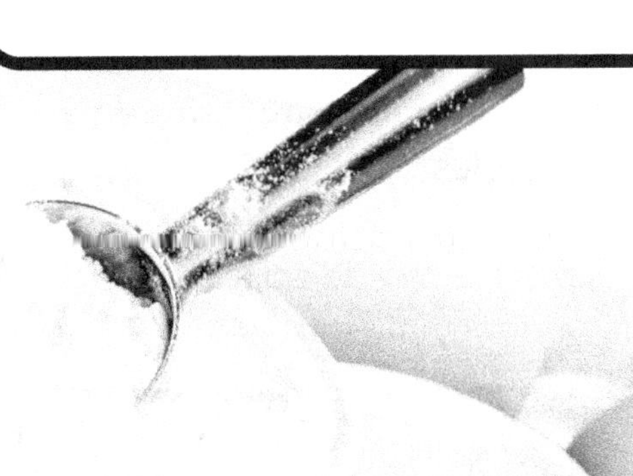

73. CLUB SANDWICHES

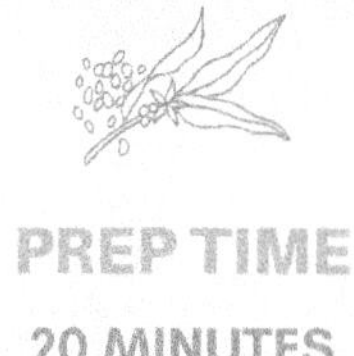

PREP TIME
20 MINUTES

COOK TIME
30 MINUTES

INGREDIENTS :

- 6 slices of toasted bread (white, wheat, or sourdough)
- 6 slices of cooked bacon
- 6 slices of turkey or ham
- 2 slices of tomato
- 2 leaves of lettuce
- 2 tbsp mayonnaise
- Salt and pepper to taste

PROCEDURE :

1. Toast the 6 slices of bread until golden brown.

2. Lay 3 of the toasted bread slices on a clean surface.

3. Spread 1 tbsp of mayonnaise on each of the 3 bread slices.

4. Layer 2 slices of bacon, 2 slices of turkey or ham, 1 slice of tomato, and 1 leaf of lettuce on each of the 3 bread slices.

5. Top each sandwich with another slice of toasted bread.

6. Repeat the layering process with the remaining ingredients to create 3 complete club sandwiches.

7. Cut each sandwich in half diagonally to serve.

Tips for Young Chefs:
- Let them measure and assemble the sandwiches themselves.

- Encourage them to experiment with different types of meat or vegetables.

- Suggest they get creative by adding a slice of cheese or a drizzle of honey mustard.

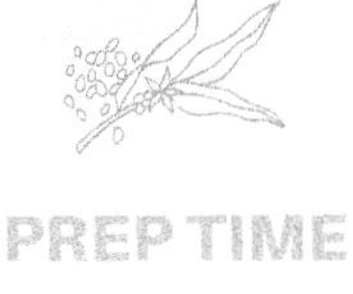

74. TUNA MELT

PREP TIME
20 MINUTES

COOK TIME
30 MINUTES

INGREDIENTS:

- 1 (5 oz) can of tuna, drained
- 2 tbsp mayonnaise
- 1 tbsp finely chopped onion (optional)
- 1 tbsp finely chopped celery (optional)
- Salt and pepper to taste
- 4 slices of bread
- 4 slices of cheddar or American cheese

PROCEDURE:

1. In a small bowl, mix together the drained tuna, mayonnaise, onion (if using), and celery (if using). Season with salt and pepper to taste.

2. Preheat a skillet or griddle over medium heat.

3. Place 4 slices of bread on a clean surface. Divide the tuna salad evenly among the 4 slices, spreading it to the edges.

4. Top each tuna•covered slice with a slice of cheese.

5. Place the sandwiches in the preheated skillet or griddle. Cook for 2•3 minutes per side, or until the bread is golden brown and the cheese is melted.

6. Carefully remove the tuna melts from the heat and let cool for a minute before serving.

Tips for Young Chefs:

• Let them measure and mix the tuna salad ingredients themselves.

• Encourage them to experiment with different types of cheese or add•ins like pickles or tomatoes.

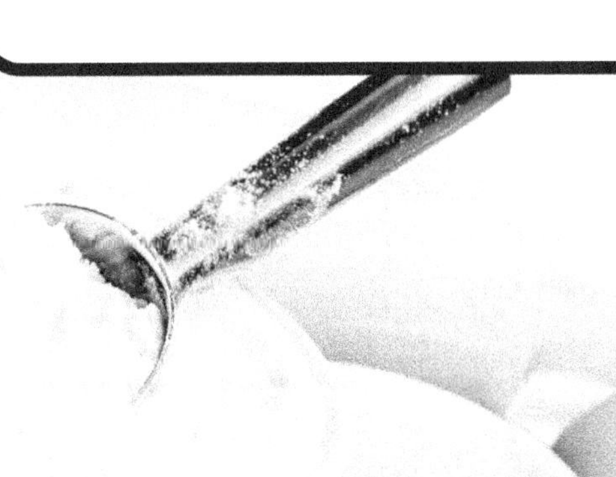

75. EGG SALAD SANDWICHES

INGREDIENTS:

- 6 hard•boiled eggs, peeled and chopped
- 2 tbsp mayonnaise
- 1 tsp Dijon mustard
- 1 tbsp finely chopped celery (optional)
- 1 tbsp finely chopped onion (optional)
- Salt and pepper to taste
- 8 slices of bread (white, wheat, or sourdough)
- Lettuce leaves (optional)

PROCEDURE:

1. In a medium bowl, gently mix together the chopped hard•boiled eggs, mayonnaise, Dijon mustard, celery (if using), and onion (if using). Season with salt and pepper to taste.

2. Lay 4 slices of bread on a clean surface.

3. Divide the egg salad mixture evenly among the 4 bread slices, spreading it to the edges.

4. If desired, top each egg salad•covered slice with a lettuce leaf.

5. Place the remaining 4 slices of bread on top to create 4 complete egg salad sandwiches.

Tips for Young Chefs:
- Let them measure and mix the egg salad ingredients themselves.

- Encourage them to experiment with different add•ins like chopped pickles or dill.

- Suggest they get creative by using different types of bread or serving the egg salad on crackers.

- Provide supervision when handling the hard•boiled eggs and chopping the vegetables.

76. GRILLED VEGGIE SANDWICHES

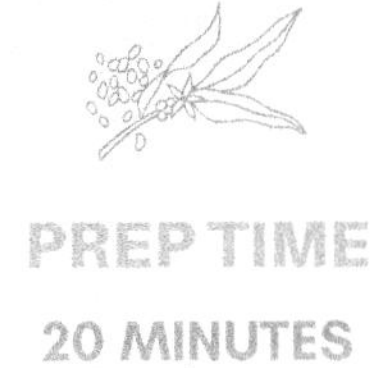

PREP TIME
20 MINUTES

COOK TIME
30 MINUTES

INGREDIENTS:

- 8 slices of whole wheat or sourdough bread
- 1 zucchini, sliced into 1/4•inch thick rounds
- 1 red bell pepper, sliced into 1/4•inch thick strips
- 1 portobello mushroom cap, sliced
- 1 cup baby spinach leaves
- 4 slices of provolone or mozzarella cheese
- 2 tbsp olive oil
- Salt and pepper to taste

Tips for Young Chefs:

- Let them measure and add the ingredients themselves.

- Encourage them to experiment with different vegetable combinations.

PROCEDURE:

1. Preheat a grill pan or outdoor grill to medium•high heat.

2. Brush the zucchini, bell pepper, and mushroom slices with the olive oil and season with salt and pepper.

3. Grill the vegetables for 2•3 minutes per side, until they are tender and have grill marks.

4. Place 4 slices of bread on a clean surface. Top each slice with a slice of cheese, some grilled vegetables, and a handful of spinach leaves.

5. Top with the remaining 4 slices of bread to make 4 sandwiches.

6. Carefully place the sandwiches on the hot grill pan or outdoor grill. Cook for 2•3 minutes per side, or until the bread is toasted and the cheese is melted.

7. Remove the sandwiches from the grill and let cool for a minute before serving.

Enjoy your delicious grilled veggie sandwiches!

77. CHICKEN CAESAR WRAPS

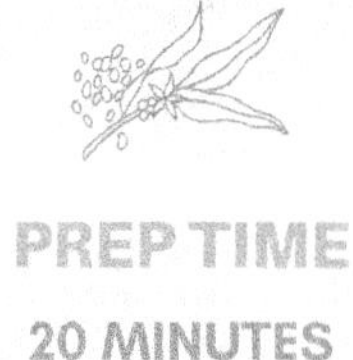 

PREP TIME
20 MINUTES

COOK TIME
30 MINUTES

INGREDIENTS :

- 2 cups cooked, shredded chicken
- 1/2 cup Caesar salad dressing
- 4 large flour tortillas or wraps
- 2 cups chopped romaine lettuce
- 1/2 cup grated Parmesan cheese
- 1/2 cup croutons

Tips for Young Chefs:

- Let them measure and assemble the wraps themselves.

- Encourage them to experiment with different types of lettuce or add•ins like diced tomatoes or sliced avocado.

- Suggest they get creative by using different types of tortillas or wraps, such as spinach or whole wheat.

PROCEDURE :

1. In a medium bowl, mix the shredded chicken and Caesar salad dressing until the chicken is well coated.

2. Lay the 4 tortillas or wraps on a clean surface.

3. Divide the chopped romaine lettuce evenly among the 4 wraps, placing it in the center.

4. Top the lettuce with the Caesar•coated chicken, spreading it out in an even layer.

5. Sprinkle the Parmesan cheese and croutons over the chicken.

6. Fold the bottom of the wrap up over the filling, then fold in the sides and continue rolling up tightly to enclose the filling.

7. Slice the wraps in half diagonally, if desired, and serve.

Enjoy your homemade chicken Caesar wraps!

78. PULLED PORK SANDWICHES

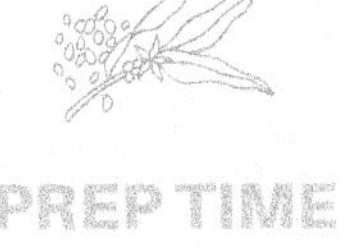

PREP TIME
20 MINUTES

COOK TIME
30 MINUTES

INGREDIENTS:

• 1 lb boneless pork shoulder or butt, cut into 2•inch cubes
• 1 cup barbecue sauce
• 4 hamburger buns or slider rolls
• Coleslaw (optional)

PROCEDURE:

1. Place the pork cubes in a slow cooker and pour the barbecue sauce over the top. Stir to coat the pork.

2. Cover the slow cooker and cook on low for 6•8 hours, or until the pork is very tender and easily shreds with a fork.

3. Once the pork is cooked, use two forks to shred the meat right in the slow cooker, mixing it with the sauce.

4. Divide the pulled pork evenly among the 4 hamburger buns or slider rolls.

5. If desired, top the pulled pork with a spoonful of coleslaw.

Tips for Young Chefs:
• Let them measure and assemble the sandwiches themselves.

• Encourage them to experiment with different barbecue sauce flavors.

• Suggest they get creative by adding pickles, onions, or other favorite toppings.

• Provide supervision when using the slow cooker and shredding the pork.

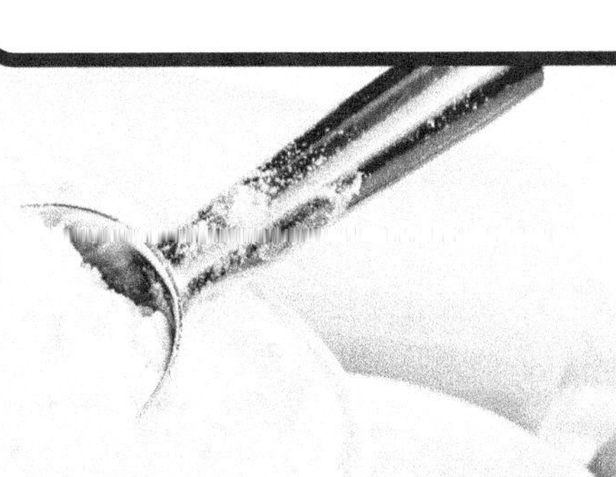

79. MEATBALL SUBS

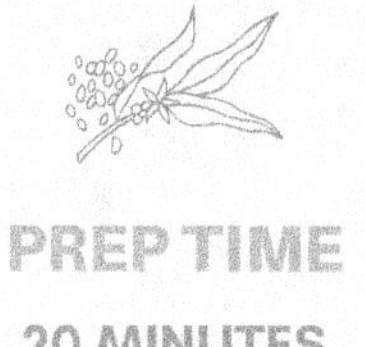

PREP TIME	**COOK TIME**
20 MINUTES	30 MINUTES

INGREDIENTS:

• 12 frozen pre•cooked meatballs
• 1 cup marinara sauce
• 4 sub or hoagie rolls, split lengthwise
• 1 cup shredded mozzarella cheese

Tips for Young Chefs:

• Let them measure and assemble the subs themselves.

• Encourage them to experiment with different types of cheese or add•ins like sliced peppers or onions.

• Suggest they get creative by making mini meatball sliders instead of full•size subs.

• Provide supervision when using the oven and handling hot cookware.

PROCEDURE:

1. Preheat your oven to 350°F (175°C).

2. In a medium saucepan, heat the marinara sauce over medium heat until simmering.

3. Add the frozen meatballs to the sauce and stir gently to coat them. Simmer for 5•7 minutes, or until the meatballs are heated through.

4. Place the split sub rolls on a baking sheet. Spoon the meatballs and sauce evenly into the rolls.

5. Top each meatball sub with the shredded mozzarella cheese.

6. Bake the meatball subs in the preheated oven for 5•7 minutes, or until the cheese is melted and bubbly.

7. Carefully remove the meatball subs from the oven and let cool for a minute before serving.

Enjoy your delicious homemade meatball subs!

80. CAPRESE SANDWICHES

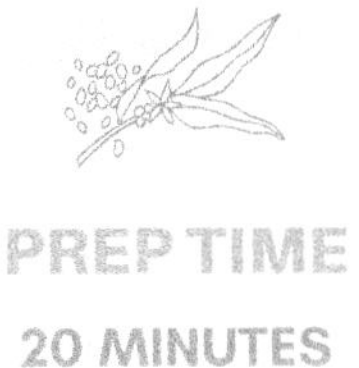

PREP TIME
20 MINUTES

COOK TIME
30 MINUTES

INGREDIENTS:

- 8 slices of fresh mozzarella cheese
- 8 slices of tomato
- 8 fresh basil leaves
- 4 ciabatta rolls or slices of crusty bread
- 2 tbsp balsamic glaze
- 2 tbsp olive oil
- Salt and pepper to taste

PROCEDURE:

1. Slice the ciabatta rolls in half horizontally to create 4 sandwiches.

2. On the bottom half of each roll, layer 2 slices of mozzarella cheese, 2 slices of tomato, and 2 fresh basil leaves.

3. Drizzle a small amount of balsamic glaze and olive oil over the caprese layers.

4. Season with a pinch of salt and pepper.

5. Place the top half of the roll on each sandwich.

Tips for Young Chefs:
- Let them assemble the sandwiches themselves.

- Encourage them to experiment with different types of bread or add•ins like pesto or balsamic vinegar.

- Suggest they get creative by making mini caprese skewers or salads instead of sandwiches.

- Provide supervision when handling the sharp knife for slicing the tomatoes and mozzarella.

Enjoy your fresh and flavorful caprese sandwiches!

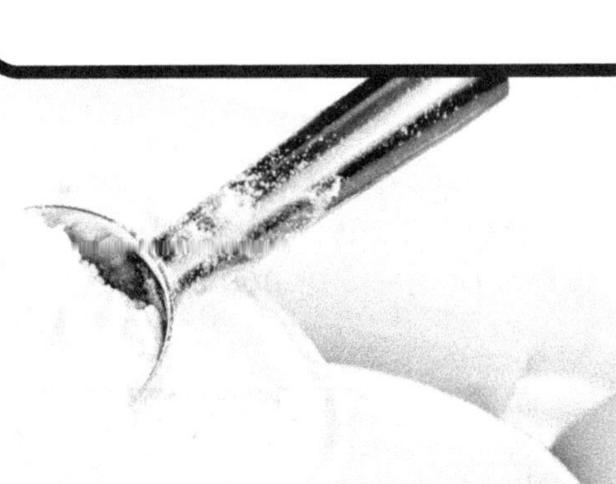

81. PASTA PRIMAVERA

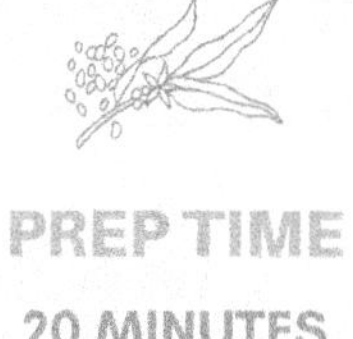 

PREP TIME
20 MINUTES

COOK TIME
30 MINUTES

INGREDIENTS:

- 8 oz penne or farfalle pasta
- 1 cup broccoli florets
- 1 cup sliced zucchini
- 1 cup sliced yellow squash
- 1 cup cherry tomatoes, halved
- 2 cloves garlic, minced
- 2 tbsp olive oil
- 1/4 cup grated Parmesan cheese
- 2 tbsp chopped fresh basil (or 1 tsp dried basil)
- Salt and pepper to taste

PROCEDURE:

1. Bring a large pot of salted water to a boil. Add the pasta and cook according to package instructions until al dente. Drain and set aside.

2. In a large skillet, heat the olive oil over medium heat. Add the garlic and sauté for 1 minute until fragrant.

3. Add the broccoli, zucchini, and yellow squash to the skillet. Sauté for 5•7 minutes, stirring occasionally, until the vegetables are tender•crisp.

4. Add the cooked pasta, cherry tomatoes, Parmesan cheese, and basil to the skillet. Toss everything together until well combined.

5. Season with salt and pepper to taste.

6. Serve the pasta primavera warm, garnished with extra Parmesan cheese and basil, if desired.

Tips for Young Chefs:

• Let them measure and add the ingredients themselves.

• Encourage them to experiment with different vegetables, such as bell peppers or asparagus.

82. FETTUCCINE ALFREDO

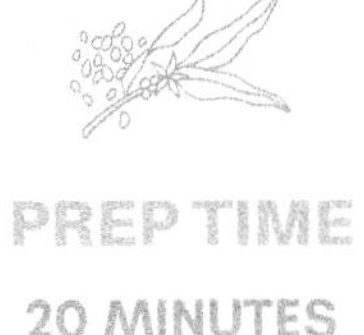 

INGREDIENTS:

- 8 oz fettuccine pasta
- 4 tbsp unsalted butter
- 1 cup heavy cream
- 1 cup grated Parmesan cheese
- 1/4 tsp salt
- 1/8 tsp black pepper

Tips for Young Chefs:

- Let them measure and add the ingredients themselves.

- Encourage them to taste the sauce and adjust the seasoning if needed.

- Suggest they get creative by adding grilled chicken or sautéed vegetables to the dish.

- Provide supervision when using the stove and handling hot cookware.

PROCEDURE:

1. Bring a large pot of salted water to a boil. Add the fettuccine and cook according to package instructions until al dente, about 8•10 minutes. Drain the pasta and set aside.

2. In a large skillet, melt the butter over medium heat.

3. Slowly pour in the heavy cream and whisk constantly until the mixture starts to thicken, about 2•3 minutes.

4. Remove the skillet from the heat and stir in the Parmesan cheese, salt, and pepper until the cheese is melted and the sauce is smooth.

5. Add the cooked fettuccine to the sauce and toss to coat the noodles evenly.

6. Serve the fettuccine alfredo immediately, garnished with extra Parmesan cheese if desired.

Enjoy your homemade fettuccine alfredo!

83. PESTO PASTA

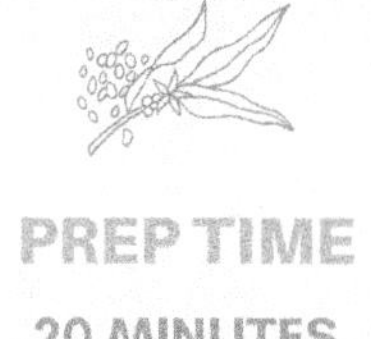 

PREP TIME
20 MINUTES

COOK TIME
30 MINUTES

INGREDIENTS :

• 8 oz pasta (such as penne, fusilli, or spaghetti)
• 1 cup fresh basil leaves
• 2 cloves garlic
• 1/4 cup pine nuts or walnuts
• 1/2 cup grated Parmesan cheese
• 1/4 cup olive oil
• 1/4 tsp salt
• 1/8 tsp black pepper

PROCEDURE :

1. Bring a large pot of salted water to a boil. Add the pasta and cook according to the package instructions until al dente. Drain the pasta and set it aside.

2. In a food processor or blender, combine the fresh basil leaves, garlic, pine nuts or walnuts, Parmesan cheese, olive oil, salt, and pepper. Blend until a smooth pesto sauce forms.

3. In a large bowl, toss the cooked pasta with the pesto sauce until the pasta is evenly coated.

4. Serve the pesto pasta warm, garnished with extra Parmesan cheese and a drizzle of olive oil, if desired.

Tips for Young Chefs:

• Let them measure and add the ingredients to the food processor or blender.

• Encourage them to experiment with different types of nuts or greens (like spinach or arugula) in the pesto.

• Suggest they get creative by adding grilled chicken or roasted vegetables to the pasta.

84. BAKED MAC AND CHEESE

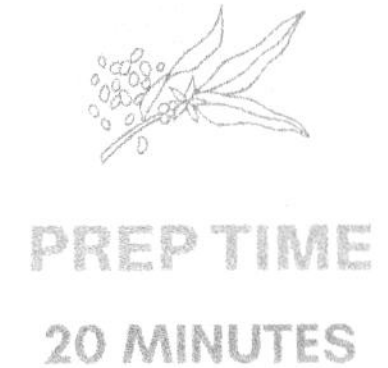

PREP TIME
20 MINUTES

COOK TIME
30 MINUTES

INGREDIENTS :

- 8 oz elbow macaroni
- 2 tbsp unsalted butter
- 2 tbsp all•purpose flour
- 2 cups milk
- 2 cups shredded cheddar cheese
- 1/2 cup grated Parmesan cheese
- 1/4 tsp salt
- 1/8 tsp black pepper

Tips for Young Chefs:
• Let them measure and add the ingredients themselves.

• Encourage them to experiment with different types of cheese or add•ins like diced ham or broccoli.

• Suggest they get creative by making individual servings in ramekins or muffin tins.

• Provide supervision when using the stove and oven.

PROCEDURE :

1. Preheat your oven to 375°F (190°C).

2. Bring a large pot of salted water to a boil. Add the elbow macaroni and cook according to the package instructions until al dente. Drain the pasta and set it aside.

3. In a medium saucepan, melt the butter over medium heat. Whisk in the flour and cook for 1 minute, stirring constantly.

4. Gradually whisk in the milk and continue cooking, stirring frequently, until the sauce thickens, about 5 minutes.

5. Remove the saucepan from the heat and stir in 1 1/2 cups of the cheddar cheese and the Parmesan cheese. Season with salt and pepper.

6. Add the cooked macaroni to the cheese sauce and stir to combine.

7. Transfer the mac and cheese to a baking dish and top with the remaining 1/2 cup of cheddar cheese.

8. Bake the mac and cheese in the preheated oven for 20•25 minutes, or until the top is golden brown and bubbly. Let the baked mac and cheese cool for 5 minutes before serving.

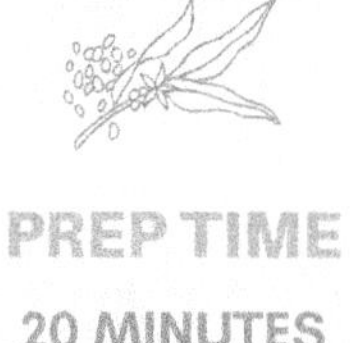

85. SPAGHETTI CARBONARA

PREP TIME
20 MINUTES

COOK TIME
30 MINUTES

INGREDIENTS:

- 8 oz spaghetti
- 4 slices of bacon, diced
- 2 eggs
- 1/2 cup grated Parmesan cheese, plus more for serving
- 2 tbsp chopped fresh parsley (optional)
- Salt and pepper to taste

Tips for Young Chefs:

- Let them measure and add the ingredients themselves.

- Encourage them to be careful when handling the hot skillet and tossing the pasta with the egg mixture.

- Suggest they get creative by adding peas or diced ham to the dish.

PROCEDURE:

1. Bring a large pot of salted water to a boil. Add the spaghetti and cook according to the package instructions until al dente. Drain the pasta, reserving 1/2 cup of the cooking water.

2. In a skillet, cook the diced bacon over medium heat until crispy, about 5•7 minutes. Drain the bacon on a paper towel•lined plate.

3. In a medium bowl, whisk together the 2 eggs and 1/2 cup of Parmesan cheese.

4. Add the cooked spaghetti to the skillet with the bacon. Toss to combine.

5. Remove the skillet from the heat and quickly pour the egg•Parmesan mixture over the hot pasta, tossing constantly to coat the noodles. The residual heat from the pasta will cook the eggs and create a creamy sauce.

6. If the sauce seems too thick, add a splash of the reserved pasta cooking water to thin it out.

7. Season the spaghetti carbonara with salt and pepper to taste.

8. Serve the spaghetti carbonara immediately, garnished with additional Parmesan cheese and chopped parsley, if desired.

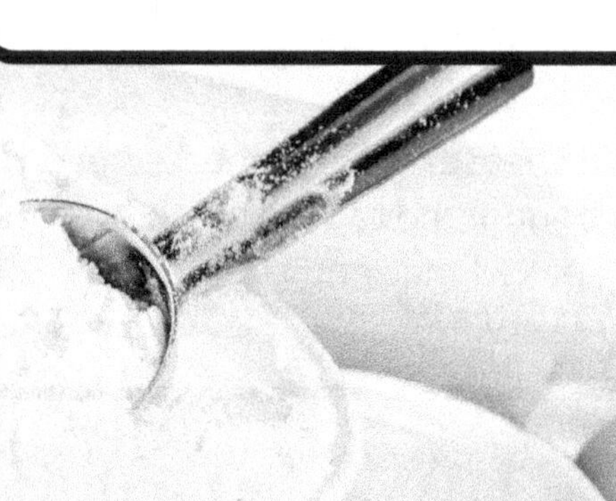

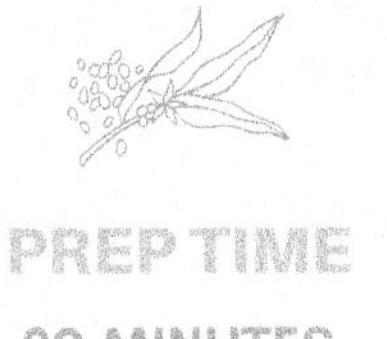

86. LASAGNA

PREP TIME
20 MINUTES

COOK TIME
30 MINUTES

INGREDIENTS:

- 8 oz lasagna noodles
- 1 lb ground beef or Italian sausage
- 1 jar (24 oz) marinara sauce
- 1 container (15 oz) ricotta cheese
- 2 cups shredded mozzarella cheese
- 1/2 cup grated Parmesan cheese
- 1 egg
- 2 tbsp chopped fresh parsley (optional)
- Salt and pepper to taste

9. Bake the lasagna in the preheated oven for 30•35 minutes, or until the cheese is melted and bubbly.

10. Let the lasagna cool for 10•15 minutes before serving.

PROCEDURE:

1. Preheat your oven to 375°F (190°C).

2. Bring a large pot of salted water to a boil. Add the lasagna noodles and cook according to the package instructions until al dente. Drain the noodles and set them aside.

3. In a large skillet, cook the ground beef or Italian sausage over medium heat until browned and crumbled. Drain any excess fat. Stir the marinara sauce into the cooked meat. Simmer for 5 minutes.

4. In a medium bowl, mix together the ricotta cheese, 1 cup of the mozzarella cheese, the Parmesan cheese, egg, and parsley (if using). Season with salt and pepper. Spread 1 cup of the meat sauce in the bottom of a 9x13•inch baking dish.

5. Layer 3•4 lasagna noodles over the sauce, then top with half of the ricotta cheese mixture and 1 cup of the meat sauce.

6. Repeat the noodle, ricotta, and meat sauce layers. Top with the remaining lasagna noodles and the remaining meat sauce. Sprinkle the remaining 1 cup of mozzarella cheese over the top.

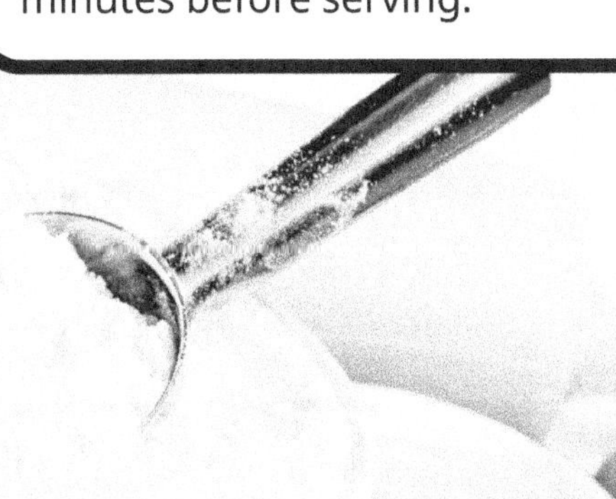

87. PASTA WITH MARINARA SAUCE

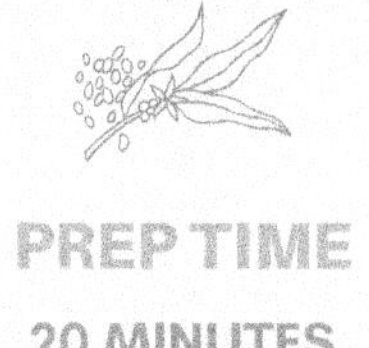

PREP TIME
20 MINUTES

COOK TIME
30 MINUTES

INGREDIENTS:

• 8 oz pasta (such as spaghetti, penne, or fusilli)
• 1 jar (24 oz) marinara sauce
• 1/4 cup grated Parmesan cheese (optional)
• Fresh basil leaves (optional)

Tips for Young Chefs:
• Let them measure and add the ingredients themselves.

• Encourage them to experiment with different types of pasta or marinara sauce flavors.

• Suggest they get creative by adding sautéed vegetables, such as mushrooms or bell peppers, to the sauce.

• Provide supervision when handling the hot cookware and draining the pasta.

PROCEDURE:

1. Bring a large pot of salted water to a boil. Add the pasta and cook according to the package instructions until al dente.

2. Drain the cooked pasta, reserving about 1/4 cup of the cooking water.

3. In a medium saucepan, heat the marinara sauce over medium heat, stirring occasionally, until it's hot and bubbly.

4. Add the cooked pasta to the saucepan with the marinara sauce. Toss the pasta to coat it evenly with the sauce, adding a splash of the reserved cooking water if the sauce seems too thick.

5. Serve the pasta with marinara sauce immediately, garnished with grated Parmesan cheese and fresh basil leaves, if desired.

Enjoy your homemade pasta with marinara sauce!

88. STUFFED SHELLS

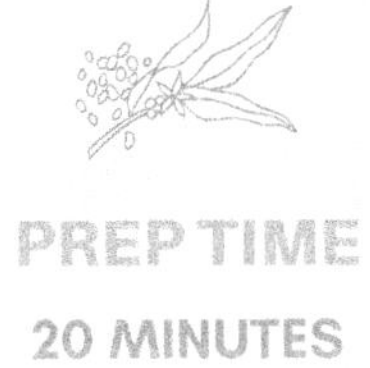

INGREDIENTS:

- 12 jumbo pasta shells
- 1 cup ricotta cheese
- 1 cup shredded mozzarella cheese, divided
- 1/4 cup grated Parmesan cheese
- 1 egg
- 2 tbsp chopped fresh parsley
- 1/4 tsp salt
- 1/8 tsp black pepper
- 1 jar (24 oz) marinara sauce

Tips for Young Chefs:
- Let them measure and stuff the pasta shells themselves.

- Encourage them to experiment with different cheese combinations or add•ins like spinach or diced tomatoes.

- Suggest they get creative by making mini stuffed shells in a muffin tin.

PROCEDURE:

1. Preheat your oven to 375°F (190°C).

2. Bring a large pot of salted water to a boil. Add the jumbo pasta shells and cook according to the package instructions until al dente. Drain the shells and set them aside.

3. In a medium bowl, mix together the ricotta cheese, 1/2 cup of the mozzarella cheese, the Parmesan cheese, egg, parsley, salt, and pepper until well combined.

4. Spread 1/2 cup of the marinara sauce in the bottom of a 9x13•inch baking dish.

5. Carefully stuff each cooked pasta shell with a spoonful of the ricotta cheese mixture, then place the stuffed shells in the baking dish in a single layer.

6. Pour the remaining marinara sauce over the top of the stuffed shells. Sprinkle the remaining 1/2 cup of mozzarella cheese over the top.

8. Bake the stuffed shells in the preheated oven for 20•25 minutes, or until the cheese is melted and bubbly. Let the stuffed shells cool for 5 minutes before serving.

89. PASTA WITH PESTO AND SUN•DRIED TOMATOES

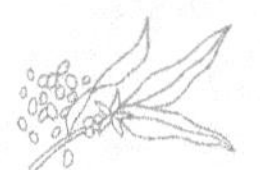

PREP TIME
20 MINUTES

COOK TIME
30 MINUTES

INGREDIENTS:

- 8 oz pasta (such as penne, fusilli, or linguine)
- 1/2 cup prepared basil pesto
- 1/2 cup chopped sun•dried tomatoes
- 1/4 cup toasted pine nuts or walnuts (optional)
- 1/4 cup grated Parmesan cheese
- Salt and pepper to taste

Tips for Young Chefs:
- Let them measure and add the ingredients themselves.

- Encourage them to experiment with different types of pasta or pesto flavors.

- Suggest they get creative by adding grilled chicken or roasted vegetables to the dish.

PROCEDURE:

1. Bring a large pot of salted water to a boil. Add the pasta and cook according to the package instructions until al dente. Drain the pasta and set it aside.

2. In a large bowl, combine the cooked pasta, basil pesto, and chopped sun•dried tomatoes. Toss to coat the pasta evenly.

3. If using, stir in the toasted pine nuts or walnuts.

4. Sprinkle the grated Parmesan cheese over the top of the pasta.

5. Season with salt and pepper to taste.

6. Serve the pasta with pesto and sun•dried tomatoes warm, garnished with extra Parmesan cheese if desired.

Enjoy your homemade pasta with pesto and sun•dried tomatoes!

90. PASTA WITH BUTTER AND PARMESAN

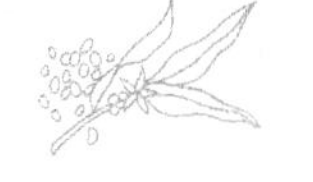

PREP TIME
20 MINUTES

COOK TIME
30 MINUTES

INGREDIENTS:

• 8 oz pasta (such as spaghetti, penne, or fusilli)
• 4 tbsp unsalted butter
• 1/2 cup grated Parmesan cheese
• Salt and pepper to taste

Tips for Young Chefs:
• Let them measure and add the ingredients themselves.

• Encourage them to experiment with different types of pasta or cheeses.

• Suggest they get creative by adding chopped fresh herbs, such as basil or parsley, or a sprinkle of red pepper flakes.

• Provide supervision when handling the hot cookware and draining the pasta.

PROCEDURE:

1. Bring a large pot of salted water to a boil. Add the pasta and cook according to the package instructions until al dente.

2. Drain the cooked pasta, reserving about 1/4 cup of the cooking water.

3. In the same pot, melt the 4 tablespoons of butter over medium heat.

4. Add the drained pasta back to the pot with the melted butter. Toss the pasta to coat it evenly with the butter.

5. Gradually add the grated Parmesan cheese, tossing the pasta continuously to incorporate the cheese. If the pasta seems too dry, add a splash of the reserved cooking water to help the cheese and butter create a creamy sauce.

6. Season the pasta with salt and pepper to taste.

7. Serve the pasta with butter and Parmesan immediately, garnished with extra Parmesan cheese if desired.

Enjoy your simple and delicious pasta with butter and Parmesan!

91. QUINOA SALAD

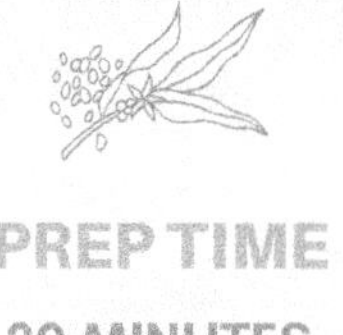

PREP TIME
20 MINUTES

COOK TIME
30 MINUTES

INGREDIENTS:

- 1 cup uncooked quinoa, rinsed
- 2 cups vegetable or chicken broth
- 1 cup diced cucumber
- 1 cup cherry tomatoes, halved
- 1/2 cup diced red onion
- 1/2 cup crumbled feta cheese
- 2 tbsp chopped fresh parsley
- 2 tbsp olive oil
- 2 tbsp lemon juice
- 1 tsp Dijon mustard
- Salt and pepper to taste

Tips for Young Chefs:

- Let them measure and add the ingredients to the bowl.

- Encourage them to experiment with different vegetables or herbs.
- Suggest they get creative by adding grilled chicken or roasted chickpeas for extra protein.

PROCEDURE:

1. In a medium saucepan, combine the rinsed quinoa and broth. Bring to a boil, then reduce heat to low, cover, and simmer for 15•20 minutes, or until the quinoa is cooked and the liquid is absorbed.

2. Transfer the cooked quinoa to a large bowl and let it cool slightly.

3. Add the diced cucumber, cherry tomatoes, red onion, feta cheese, and chopped parsley to the bowl with the quinoa.

4. In a small bowl, whisk together the olive oil, lemon juice, and Dijon mustard. Pour the dressing over the quinoa salad and toss to coat.

5. Season the quinoa salad with salt and pepper to taste.

6. Serve the quinoa salad chilled or at room temperature.

Enjoy your refreshing and nutritious quinoa salad!

92. STUFFED ZUCCHINI BOATS

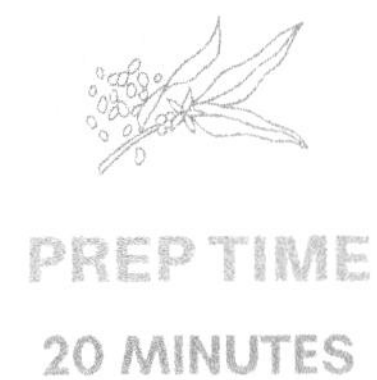

PREP TIME
20 MINUTES

COOK TIME
30 MINUTES

INGREDIENTS:

- 3 medium zucchini, halved lengthwise
- 1/2 lb ground turkey or ground beef
- 1/2 cup cooked rice
- 1/4 cup diced onion
- 1 clove garlic, minced
- 1/2 cup shredded mozzarella cheese
- 2 tbsp grated Parmesan cheese
- 1 tsp dried oregano
- Salt and pepper to taste

Tips for Young Chefs:

- Let them scoop out the zucchini flesh and mix the filling ingredients.

- Encourage them to experiment with different fillings, such as adding diced tomatoes or spinach.

PROCEDURE:

1. Preheat your oven to 375°F (190°C).

2. Using a spoon, scoop out the flesh from the center of each zucchini half, leaving about 1/4 inch of the zucchini shell. Chop the scooped•out zucchini flesh.

3. In a skillet, cook the ground turkey or beef over medium heat until browned and crumbled. Drain any excess fat.

4. Add the chopped zucchini flesh, cooked rice, onion, and garlic to the skillet. Cook for 5 minutes, stirring occasionally, until the vegetables are tender.

5. Remove the skillet from the heat and stir in the mozzarella cheese, Parmesan cheese, and oregano. Season with salt and pepper to taste.

6. Arrange the zucchini boats in a baking dish. Spoon the meat and rice mixture evenly into the zucchini shells.

7. Bake the stuffed zucchini boats in the preheated oven for 20•25 minutes, or until the zucchini is tender and the filling is hot and bubbly.

8. Serve the stuffed zucchini boats warm.

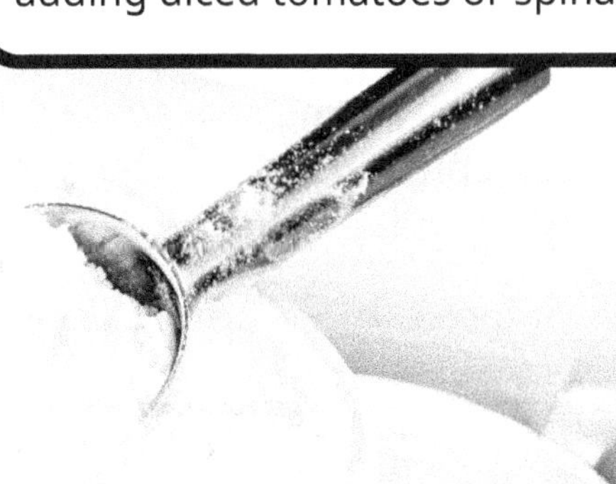

93. VEGETABLE STIR•FRY

PREP TIME
20 MINUTES

COOK TIME
30 MINUTES

INGREDIENTS:

- 2 tbsp vegetable oil
- 1 cup broccoli florets
- 1 cup sliced carrots
- 1 cup sliced bell peppers
- 1 cup sliced mushrooms
- 1 cup snow peas or snap peas
- 2 cloves garlic, minced
- 2 tbsp soy sauce
- 1 tsp sesame oil (optional)
- Salt and pepper to taste
- Cooked rice or noodles, for serving (optional)

PROCEDURE:

1. Heat the vegetable oil in a large skillet or wok over high heat.

2. Add the broccoli, carrots, bell peppers, mushrooms, and snow/snap peas to the hot pan. Stir•fry the vegetables for 5•7 minutes, or until they are tender•crisp.

3. Add the minced garlic to the pan and stir•fry for an additional 1 minute, until fragrant.

4. Pour the soy sauce and sesame oil (if using) over the vegetables and toss to coat.

5. Season the stir•fry with salt and pepper to taste.

6. Serve the vegetable stir•fry immediately, over cooked rice or noodles if desired.

Tips for Young Chefs:
- Let them measure and add the vegetables to the pan.
- Encourage them to experiment with different vegetable combinations.
- Suggest they get creative by adding cooked chicken, beef, or tofu for a protein boost.
- Provide supervision when using the hot skillet or wok.

94. GRILLED CHICKEN SALAD

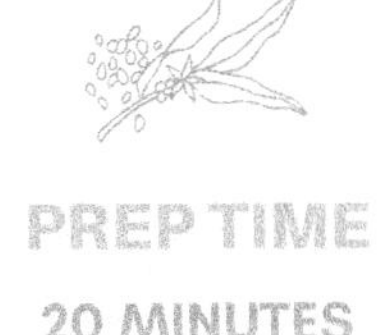 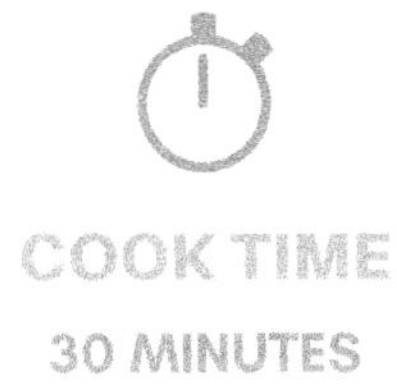

PREP TIME
20 MINUTES

COOK TIME
30 MINUTES

INGREDIENTS:

- 2 boneless, skinless chicken breasts
- 1 tbsp olive oil
- 1 tsp garlic powder
- 1 tsp dried oregano
- Salt and pepper to taste
- 4 cups mixed greens (such as romaine, spinach, arugula)
- 1 cup cherry tomatoes, halved
- 1/2 cucumber, sliced
- 1/4 red onion, thinly sliced
- 2 tbsp shredded cheddar cheese
- 2 tbsp ranch dressing or balsamic vinaigrette

PROCEDURE:

1. Preheat grill or grill pan to medium•high heat.

2. Rub the chicken breasts with olive oil and season with garlic powder, oregano, salt, and pepper.

3. Grill the chicken for 5•7 minutes per side, or until cooked through. Let cool slightly, then slice or chop the chicken.

4. In a large salad bowl, combine the mixed greens, tomatoes, cucumber, and red onion.

5. Top the salad with the grilled chicken, shredded cheese, and your choice of dressing.

6. Toss everything together and serve immediately.

This salad is a great way to get kids involved in the kitchen. They can help measure ingredients, assemble the salad, and even grill the chicken with adult supervision. Enjoy!

95. FRUIT AND YOGURT PARFAITS

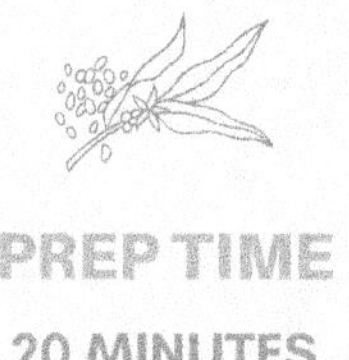 

PREP TIME
20 MINUTES

COOK TIME
30 MINUTES

INGREDIENTS :

• 2 cups plain or vanilla Greek yogurt
• 1 cup fresh or frozen berries (such as strawberries, blueberries, or raspberries)
• 1/2 cup granola or crushed graham crackers
• 2 tbsp honey (optional)

PROCEDURE :

1. In a clear glass or jar, layer the ingredients in the following order:
  • 1/4 cup of yogurt
  • 2•3 tablespoons of berries
  • 1•2 tablespoons of granola or crushed graham crackers
  • Repeat the layers until you reach the top of the glass or jar.

2. If desired, drizzle a small amount of honey over the top of the parfait.

3. Refrigerate the parfaits until ready to serve.

Tips for Young Chefs:

• Let them measure and layer the ingredients themselves.

• Encourage them to experiment with different types of fruit, yogurt, and toppings.

• Suggest they get creative by making parfaits in small jars or cups for individual servings.

• Provide supervision when handling the glass or jar, especially if it's fragile.

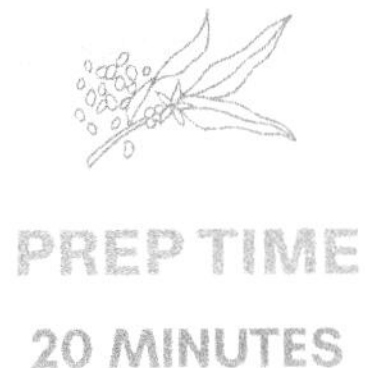

96. VEGGIE TACOS

PREP TIME
20 MINUTES

COOK TIME
30 MINUTES

INGREDIENTS :

• 1 cup diced bell peppers (any color)
• 1 cup diced onion
• 1 cup diced zucchini or yellow squash
• 1 cup canned black beans, rinsed and drained
• 1 tsp chili powder
• 1 tsp cumin
• 1/2 tsp garlic powder
• Salt and pepper to taste
• 8•10 small corn or flour tortillas
• Toppings: shredded lettuce, diced tomatoes, shredded cheese, sour cream, salsa

PROCEDURE :

1. In a large skillet, heat 1 tbsp of olive oil over medium heat. Add the diced bell peppers, onion, and zucchini. Sauté for 5•7 minutes, until the vegetables are tender.

2. Add the black beans, chili powder, cumin, garlic powder, salt, and pepper. Stir to combine and cook for another 2•3 minutes.

3. Warm the tortillas according to package instructions. You can do this in the microwave, on a dry skillet, or in the oven wrapped in foil.

4. To assemble the tacos, place a spoonful of the veggie and bean mixture into each tortilla. Top with your desired toppings like shredded lettuce, diced tomatoes, shredded cheese, sour cream, and salsa.

This is a great recipe for kids to get involved in.

• Measure and add the vegetables to the skillet
• Rinse and drain the black beans
• Sprinkle on the spices
• Assemble the tacos with their favorite toppings

The combination of flavorful veggies, protein•packed beans, and fun toppings makes these veggie tacos a hit with kids and adults alike. Enjoy!

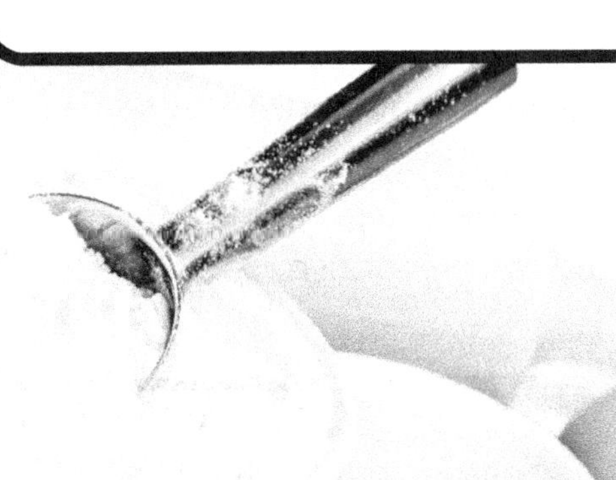

97. CAULIFLOWER RICE

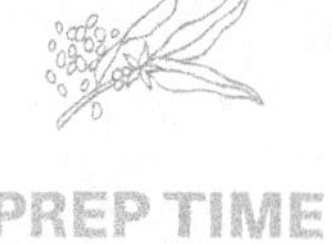 

PREP TIME	COOK TIME
20 MINUTES	30 MINUTES

INGREDIENTS:

• 1 head of cauliflower, cut into florets
• 1 tbsp olive oil
• Salt and pepper to taste

PROCEDURE:

1. Wash the cauliflower florets and pat them dry with a paper towel.

2. Place the cauliflower florets in a food processor and pulse until the cauliflower is broken down into small, rice•like pieces. Be careful not to over•process, or it will become mushy.

3. Heat the olive oil in a large skillet over medium heat.

4. Add the cauliflower rice to the skillet and cook, stirring occasionally, for 5•7 minutes, or until the cauliflower is tender and lightly browned.

5. Season with salt and pepper to taste.

That's it! Cauliflower rice is a great low•carb alternative to traditional rice, and it's super easy to make. Kids can help with the whole process, from washing the cauliflower to pulsing it in the food processor and cooking it in the skillet.

Some ideas for serving cauliflower rice:
• As a side dish, instead of regular rice
• In burrito bowls or stir•fries
• Mixed with sautéed vegetables
• Topped with grilled chicken or fish

98. BAKED SWEET POTATO FRIES

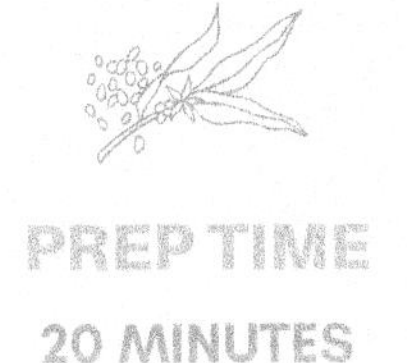

PREP TIME
20 MINUTES

COOK TIME
30 MINUTES

INGREDIENTS:

- 2 medium sweet potatoes, peeled and cut into 1/2•inch thick fry shapes
- 2 tbsp olive oil
- 1 tsp garlic powder
- 1 tsp paprika
- 1/2 tsp salt
- 1/4 tsp black pepper

This is a great recipe for kids to help with! They can:

- Wash and peel the sweet potatoes

- Cut the sweet potatoes into fry shapes (with adult supervision)
- Toss the fries with the oil and seasonings in the bowl

- Arrange the fries on the baking sheet

PROCEDURE:

1. Preheat your oven to 400°F (200°C). Line a baking sheet with parchment paper or a silicone baking mat.

2. In a large bowl, toss the sweet potato fry shapes with the olive oil, garlic powder, paprika, salt, and black pepper until they are evenly coated.

3. Spread the seasoned sweet potato fries in a single layer on the prepared baking sheet, making sure they are not touching each other.

4. Bake for 20•25 minutes, flipping the fries halfway through, until they are crispy and golden brown.

5. Remove the baked sweet potato fries from the oven and let them cool for a few minutes before serving.

Baked sweet potato fries are a healthier alternative to traditional french fries, and they're packed with vitamins and fiber. Serve them as a side dish or enjoy them as a snack. Encourage your young chefs to experiment with different seasoning blends, too!

99. CHICKEN AND VEGGIE SKEWERS

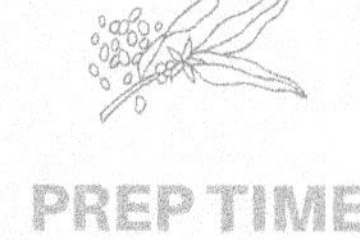

PREP TIME
20 MINUTES

COOK TIME
30 MINUTES

INGREDIENTS :

- 1 lb boneless, skinless chicken breasts, cut into 1•inch cubes
- 1 red bell pepper, cut into 1•inch pieces
- 1 zucchini, cut into 1•inch slices
- 1 red onion, cut into 1•inch pieces
- 2 tbsp olive oil
- 1 tsp dried oregano
- 1/2 tsp garlic powder
- Salt and pepper to taste
- Wooden or metal skewers

PROCEDURE :

1. If using wooden skewers, soak them in water for 30 minutes to prevent them from burning.

2. In a large bowl, combine the cubed chicken, bell pepper, zucchini, and red onion. Drizzle with the olive oil and sprinkle with the oregano, garlic powder, salt, and pepper. Toss to coat the ingredients evenly.

3. Thread the chicken and vegetables onto the skewers, alternating the ingredients.

4. Preheat your grill or grill pan to medium•high heat.

5. Grill the skewers for 12•15 minutes, turning occasionally, until the chicken is cooked through and the vegetables are tender.

6. Serve the chicken and veggie skewers hot, with any desired dipping sauces on the side.

Tips for Young Chefs:
- Let them measure and assemble the skewers themselves.
- Encourage them to experiment with different vegetables or marinades.
- Suggest they get creative by making mini skewers or using different protein options like shrimp or tofu

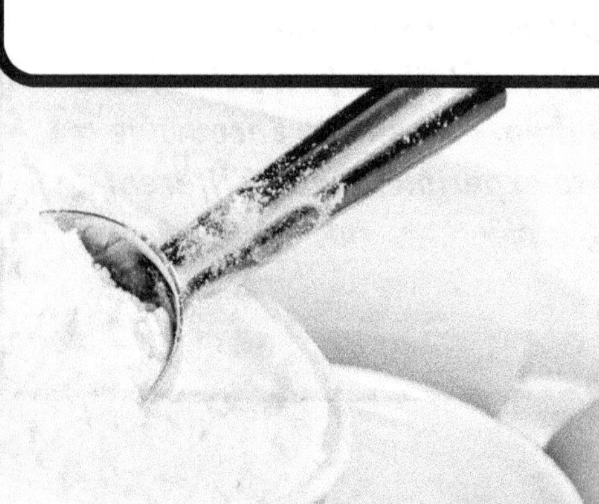

100. GREEK SALAD

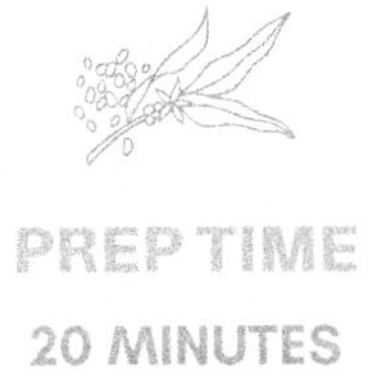

INGREDIENTS:

- 1 head of romaine lettuce, washed and chopped
- 1 cup cherry tomatoes, halved
- 1 cucumber, diced
- 1/2 red onion, thinly sliced
- 1 cup crumbled feta cheese
- 1/2 cup kalamata olives, pitted and halved
- 2 tbsp olive oil
- 1 tbsp red wine vinegar
- 1 tsp dried oregano
- 1/2 tsp salt
- 1/4 tsp black pepper

PROCEDURE:

1. In a large salad bowl, combine the chopped romaine lettuce, cherry tomatoes, diced cucumber, and sliced red onion.

2. Sprinkle the crumbled feta cheese and halved kalamata olives over the top of the salad.

3. In a small bowl, whisk together the olive oil, red wine vinegar, dried oregano, salt, and black pepper to make the dressing.

4. Just before serving, drizzle the dressing over the salad and toss gently to coat.

This Greek salad is a great way to get kids involved in the kitchen. They can:
- Wash and tear the romaine lettuce
- Halve the cherry tomatoes
- Dice the cucumber
- Slice the red onion
- Sprinkle the feta cheese and olives
- Whisk the dressing ingredients

Encourage your young chefs to taste the salad and adjust the seasoning to their liking. They can also experiment with adding other Mediterranean•inspired ingredients, like pepperoncini, chickpeas, or grilled chicken.

101. MICROWAVE MUG CAKES

PREP TIME
20 MINUTES

COOK TIME
30 MINUTES

INGREDIENTS:

- 4 tbsp all•purpose flour
- 4 tbsp sugar
- 2 tbsp cocoa powder (for chocolate mug cake)
- 1 egg
- 3 tbsp milk
- 3 tbsp vegetable oil
- 1 tsp vanilla extract
- Pinch of salt

PROCEDURE:

1. In a microwave•safe mug, whisk together the flour, sugar, and cocoa powder (if making a chocolate mug cake).

2. Add the egg, milk, vegetable oil, vanilla extract, and a pinch of salt. Stir until the batter is smooth and well combined.

3. Microwave the mug cake on high for 1•2 minutes, or until the cake is puffed up and cooked through. The timing may vary depending on your microwave, so keep an eye on it.

4. Carefully remove the mug from the microwave (it will be hot!). Allow the mug cake to cool for a minute or two before enjoying.

Tips for Young Chefs:
- Let them measure and mix the ingredients in the mug themselves.
- Encourage them to experiment with different flavors, like adding a tablespoon of peanut butter or a handful of chocolate chips.
- Suggest they get creative by topping the mug cake with whipped cream, ice cream, or a drizzle of chocolate or caramel sauce.
- Provide supervision when using the microwave, as the mug will be hot.

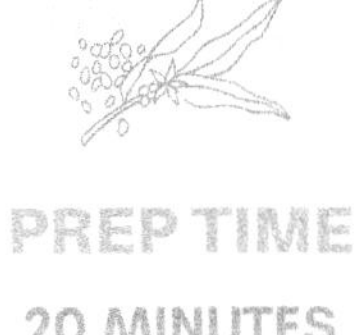

102. RAMEN NOODLES WITH VEGGIES

PREP TIME
20 MINUTES

COOK TIME
30 MINUTES

INGREDIENTS:

• 2 packages of ramen noodles (discard the seasoning packets)
• 2 cups of mixed vegetables (such as broccoli florets, sliced carrots, snow peas, and mushrooms)
• 2 cups of low•sodium vegetable or chicken broth
• 2 tbsp soy sauce
• 1 tsp sesame oil
• 1 tsp grated ginger (optional)
• 2 green onions, sliced (optional)
• Salt and pepper to taste

You can also let your young chefs choose their favorite vegetables to add to the ramen. Encourage them to try new veggies and experiment with different flavor combinations.

PROCEDURE:

1. Bring the vegetable or chicken broth to a boil in a large saucepan.

2. Add the ramen noodles and cook for 2•3 minutes, until the noodles are tender.

3. Add the mixed vegetables to the saucepan and continue cooking for another 2•3 minutes, until the vegetables are crisp•tender.

4. Stir in the soy sauce, sesame oil, and grated ginger (if using).

5. Remove the saucepan from the heat and season with salt and pepper to taste.

6. Ladle the ramen noodles and vegetables into bowls and top with the sliced green onions (if using).

This recipe is perfect for young chefs because it's easy to make and customizable. Here are some ways kids can get involved:

• Measure and add the broth, soy sauce, and sesame oil
• Break the ramen noodles into the saucepan
• Wash and chop the vegetables
• Sprinkle the green onions on top

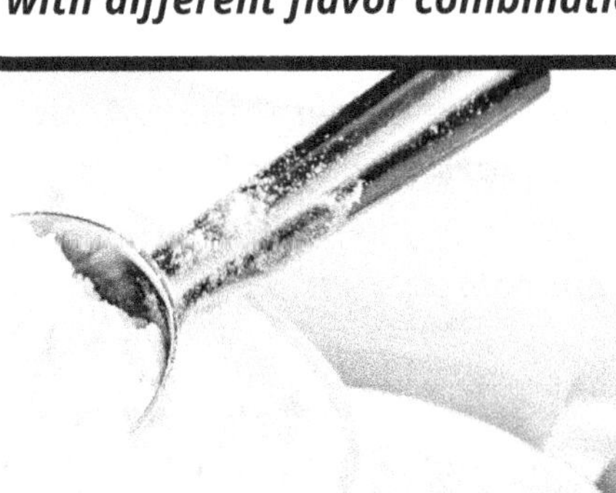

103. INSTANT OATMEAL WITH TOPPINGS

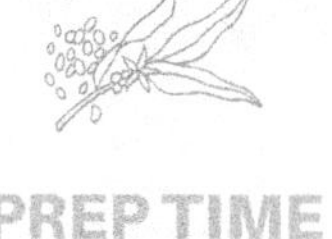

PREP TIME
20 MINUTES

COOK TIME
30 MINUTES

INGREDIENTS :

- 1 packet of instant oatmeal (plain or flavored)
- 1 cup of milk or non•dairy milk
- Toppings (choose 2•3):
  - Fresh or frozen berries (such as blueberries, raspberries, or strawberries)
  - Sliced banana
  - Chopped nuts (such as almonds or walnuts)
  - Honey or maple syrup
  - Cinnamon
  - Peanut butter or almond butter

PROCEDURE :

1. In a microwave•safe bowl, combine the instant oatmeal packet and the milk. Stir to mix well.

2. Microwave the oatmeal for 1•2 minutes, or until it's hot and cooked through. Be careful, as the bowl may be hot.

3. Carefully remove the bowl from the microwave and stir the oatmeal again.

4. Add your desired toppings to the oatmeal and stir to combine.

This recipe is perfect for young chefs because it's easy to make and customizable. Here are some ways kids can get involved:

- Measure and add the milk to the oatmeal
- Microwave the oatmeal (with adult supervision)
- Choose their favorite toppings and add them to the oatmeal
- Stir the oatmeal and toppings together

Encourage your young chefs to experiment with different toppings and flavor combinations. They can try adding fresh or frozen fruit, nuts, nut butters, honey, cinnamon, or even a sprinkle of cocoa powder for a chocolatey twist.

104. MICROWAVE NACHOS

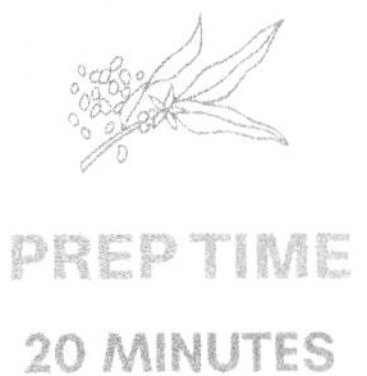

PREP TIME
20 MINUTES

COOK TIME
30 MINUTES

INGREDIENTS:

- 1 bag (9•10 oz) tortilla chips
- 1 cup shredded cheddar or Mexican blend cheese
- 1/2 cup salsa
- 2 tbsp sliced black olives (optional)
- 2 tbsp diced jalapeños (optional)
- Sour cream (optional, for serving)

PROCEDURE:

1. Arrange the tortilla chips in a single layer on a microwave•safe plate.

2. Sprinkle the shredded cheese evenly over the chips.

3. Microwave the nachos on high for 1•2 minutes, or until the cheese is melted and bubbly.

4. Carefully remove the plate from the microwave.

5. Spoon the salsa over the melted cheese, and top with the sliced black olives and diced jalapeños, if using.

6. Serve the microwave nachos immediately, with sour cream on the side if desired.

Tips for Young Chefs:
- Let them assemble the nachos on the plate and add the toppings.
- Encourage them to experiment with different chip and cheese combinations.
- Suggest they get creative by adding cooked ground beef, shredded chicken, or diced tomatoes.
- Provide supervision when using the microwave, as the plate and nachos will be hot.

105. MICROWAVE SCRAMBLED EGGS

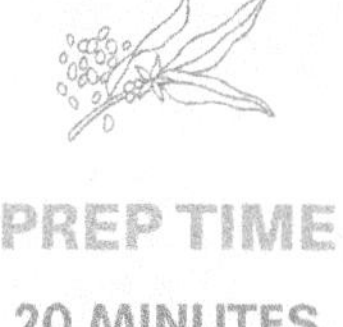

PREP TIME
20 MINUTES

COOK TIME
30 MINUTES

INGREDIENTS :

- 2 eggs
- 1 tbsp milk or water
- 1/2 tsp butter or oil
- Salt and pepper to taste

PROCEDURE :

1. Crack the 2 eggs into a microwave•safe bowl or mug. Add the milk or water and whisk the mixture together with a fork until well combined.

2. Microwave the egg mixture for 30 seconds, then remove it from the microwave and stir with a fork.

3. Microwave the eggs for another 30 seconds, then remove and stir again. Repeat this process, microwaving in 30•second intervals and stirring, until the eggs are cooked through and fluffy, about 1•2 minutes total.

4. Add the butter or oil and stir to coat the eggs. Season with salt and pepper to taste.

This is a great recipe for young chefs because:

- It's simple and easy to make
- They can crack the eggs and whisk the mixture themselves
- They can watch the eggs cook in the microwave and stir them
- They can add the butter/oil and season the eggs to their liking

Microwave scrambled eggs are a quick and easy breakfast or snack that kids can make on their own (with adult supervision). Enjoy!

106. MICROWAVE QUESADILLAS

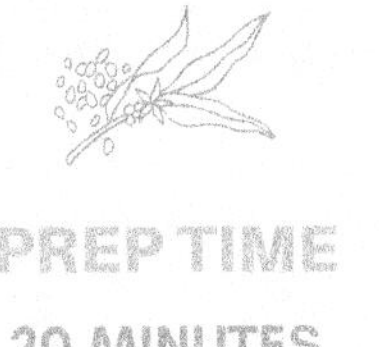

PREP TIME
20 MINUTES

COOK TIME
30 MINUTES

INGREDIENTS:

• 4 small flour tortillas
• 1 cup shredded cheese (cheddar, Monterey Jack, or a blend)
• Optional fillings: cooked chicken, black beans, diced bell peppers, onions, etc.

Encourage your young chef to get creative with the fillings. They can try adding cooked chicken, black beans, diced bell peppers, onions, or any other favorite toppings.

Microwave quesadillas are a quick and easy snack or light meal that kids can make on their own (with adult supervision). Serve them with salsa, guacamole, or sour cream for dipping. Enjoy!

PROCEDURE:

1. Lay two of the tortillas on a microwave•safe plate.

2. Sprinkle half of the shredded cheese evenly over the tortillas. If using any additional fillings, place them on top of the cheese.

3. Top each tortilla with another tortilla to create a quesadilla.

4. Microwave the quesadillas for 45 seconds to 1 minute, or until the cheese is melted and the tortillas are warm.

5. Carefully remove the quesadillas from the microwave. Use a spatula to transfer them to a cutting board.

6. Cut each quesadilla into triangles and serve warm.

This is a great recipe for young chefs because:

• It's simple and easy to assemble
• They can choose their own fillings
• They can practice using the microwave safely
• They can cut the quesadillas into triangles

107. MICROWAVE BAKED POTATOES

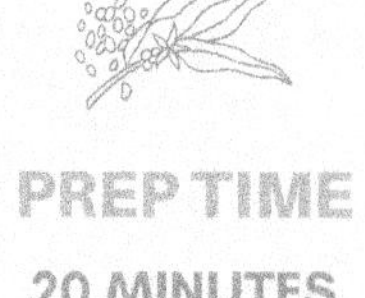

PREP TIME
20 MINUTES

COOK TIME
30 MINUTES

INGREDIENTS :

• 4 medium•sized russet potatoes, scrubbed clean
• Olive oil or vegetable oil
• Salt and pepper

Toppings (optional):
• Butter
• Sour cream
• Shredded cheese
• Chopped bacon
• Chives or green onions

Microwave baked potatoes are a quick and easy side dish or snack that kids will love. Encourage them to experiment with different toppings to find their favorite combinations.

PROCEDURE :

1. Use a fork to poke several holes all over the surface of each potato. This will allow steam to escape while cooking.

2. Rub the outside of the potatoes with a small amount of olive oil or vegetable oil. This will help the skin get crispy.

3. Place the potatoes on a microwave•safe plate or in a microwave•safe baking dish.

4. Microwave the potatoes on high for 5•7 minutes per potato, flipping them halfway through the cooking time. The potatoes are done when they are soft when squeezed.

5. Carefully remove the potatoes from the microwave. Use tongs or oven mitts, as they will be very hot.

6. Let the potatoes cool for a few minutes, then use a knife to slice them open. Fluff the insides with a fork.

7. Season the potatoes with salt and pepper to taste. Add your desired toppings, such as butter, sour cream, shredded cheese, chopped bacon, or chives.

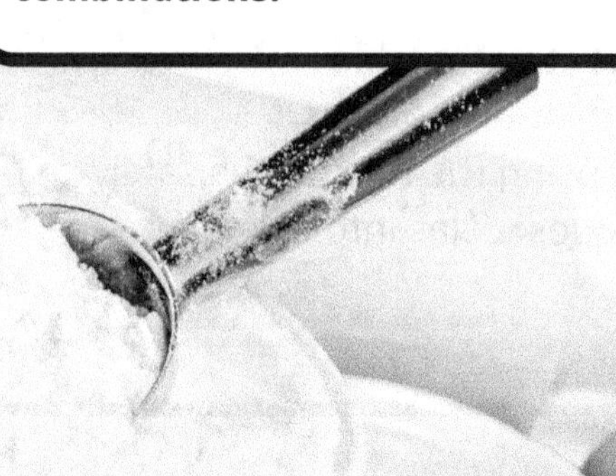

108. MICROWAVE S'MORES

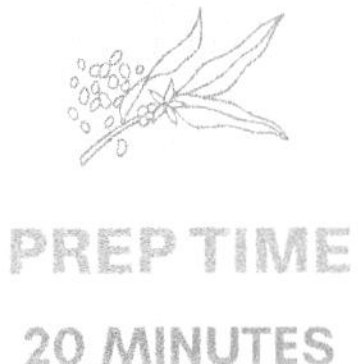

PREP TIME
20 MINUTES

COOK TIME
30 MINUTES

INGREDIENTS :

• Graham crackers
• Chocolate bars (milk chocolate or dark chocolate)
• Marshmallows

This is a great recipe for young chefs because:

• It's simple and easy to assemble

• They can choose their favorite graham crackers, chocolate, and marshmallows

• They can safely operate the microwave with adult supervision

• They can watch the marshmallow puff up in the microwave

• They get to enjoy a delicious, gooey treat!

PROCEDURE :

1. Break the graham crackers in half to create squares.

2. Place one graham cracker square on a microwave•safe plate.

3. Top the graham cracker with a piece of chocolate, then top the chocolate with a marshmallow.

4. Place another graham cracker square on top to create a s'more sandwich.

5. Microwave the s'more for 15•20 seconds, just until the marshmallow is puffed and softened.

6. Carefully remove the s'more from the microwave. The plate and s'more will be hot, so use caution.

7. Allow the s'more to cool for a minute before enjoying.

Encourage your young chef to experiment with different flavor combinations, like using dark chocolate or adding a sprinkle of cinnamon or crushed graham crackers on top.

109. MICROWAVE MAC AND CHEESE

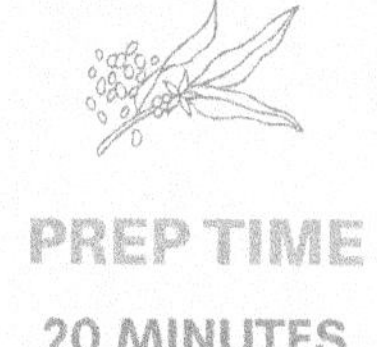 

PREP TIME
20 MINUTES

COOK TIME
30 MINUTES

INGREDIENTS:

- 1 cup uncooked elbow macaroni
- 1 cup milk
- 1/2 cup shredded cheddar cheese
- 2 tbsp butter
- 1/4 tsp salt
- 1/8 tsp black pepper

Encourage your young chef to get creative with the toppings. They can try adding diced tomatoes, cooked bacon bits, or even some frozen peas for extra nutrition.

Microwave mac and cheese is a quick and easy comfort food that kids can make on their own (with adult supervision). Enjoy!

PROCEDURE:

1. Place the uncooked macaroni in a microwave•safe bowl. Add the milk and stir to combine.

2. Microwave the macaroni and milk for 3 minutes. Carefully remove the bowl from the microwave.

3. Stir the macaroni and milk, then microwave for another 2•3 minutes, or until the macaroni is tender.

4. Carefully remove the bowl from the microwave. Add the shredded cheddar cheese, butter, salt, and pepper. Stir until the cheese is melted and the ingredients are well combined.

5. Serve the microwave mac and cheese warm.

This is a great recipe for young chefs because:

- It's simple and easy to make
- They can measure and add the ingredients to the bowl
- They can safely operate the microwave with adult supervision
- They can stir the mac and cheese and add the seasonings

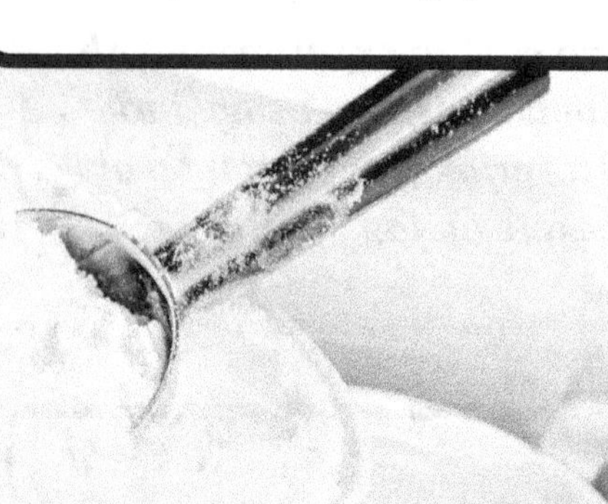

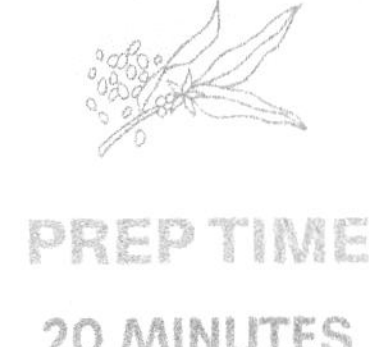

110. MICROWAVE POPCORN

PREP TIME
20 MINUTES

COOK TIME
30 MINUTES

INGREDIENTS:

• 1/4 cup unpopped popcorn kernels
• 1 tbsp olive oil or melted butter
• Salt (optional)

Equipment:
• Microwave•safe bowl with a lid or a microwave popcorn popper

Microwave popcorn is a fun and easy snack that kids can make on their own (with adult supervision, of course). Encourage them to experiment with different seasonings, such as garlic powder, chili powder, or grated Parmesan cheese.

Enjoy your freshly popped, homemade microwave popcorn!

PROCEDURE:

1. Place the unpopped popcorn kernels in the microwave•safe bowl or popcorn popper.

2. Drizzle the olive oil or melted butter over the kernels and stir to coat them evenly.

3. Cover the bowl with the lid or place the popcorn popper in the microwave.

4. Microwave the popcorn on high for 2•3 minutes, or until the popping slows to 2•3 seconds between pops.

5. Carefully remove the bowl or popper from the microwave, as it will be hot.

6. Pour the freshly popped popcorn into a serving bowl and, if desired, sprinkle with a pinch of salt.

This is a great recipe for young chefs because it's simple, quick, and they can get involved in the whole process:

• Measuring the popcorn kernels
• Drizzling and stirring in the oil or butter
• Covering the bowl or placing the popper in the microwave
• Listening for the popping to slow down
• Carefully removing the hot bowl or popper

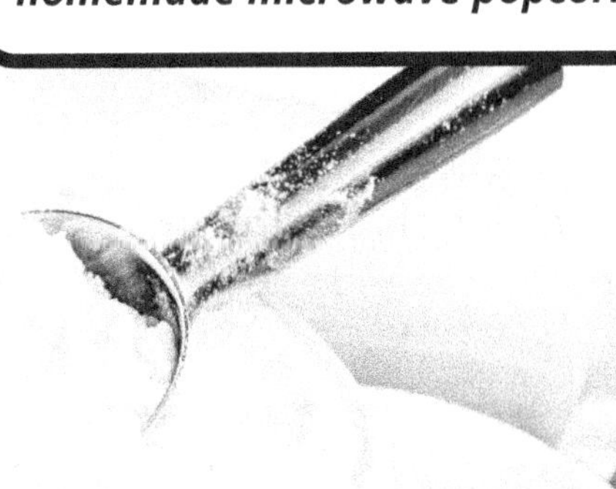

111. MINI PIZZAS

PREP TIME
20 MINUTES

COOK TIME
30 MINUTES

INGREDIENTS:

• 1 package of English muffins, split in half
• 1 cup of marinara or pizza sauce
• 1 cup of shredded mozzarella cheese
• Toppings (such as pepperoni, mushrooms, bell peppers, onions)

Encourage your young chef to get creative with the toppings. They can try different vegetables, meats, or even experiment with different types of cheese. This is a fun and interactive way for kids to make their own personalized mini pizzas.

Serve the mini pizzas warm and enjoy! This is a great snack or light meal that the whole family can enjoy.

PROCEDURE:

1. Preheat your oven to 400°F (200°C).

2. Place the split English muffin halves on a baking sheet.

3. Spoon about 2•3 tablespoons of marinara or pizza sauce onto each muffin half, spreading it to the edges.

4. Sprinkle the shredded mozzarella cheese evenly over the sauce.

5. Add any desired toppings, such as pepperoni, mushrooms, bell peppers, or onions.

6. Bake the mini pizzas in the preheated oven for 8•10 minutes, or until the cheese is melted and bubbly.

7. Carefully remove the mini pizzas from the oven and let them cool for a few minutes before serving.

This is a great recipe for young chefs because:

• It's easy to assemble and customize
• They can help measure and spread the sauce
• They can sprinkle the cheese and add their favorite toppings

112. HOMEMADE DONUTS

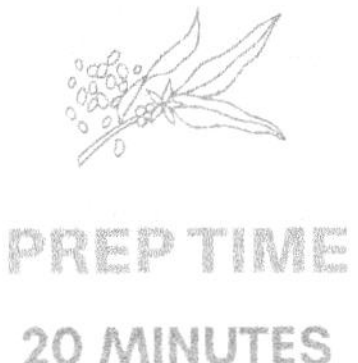

PREP TIME
20 MINUTES

COOK TIME
30 MINUTES

INGREDIENTS:

- 2 cups all•purpose flour
- 1/4 cup granulated sugar
- 2 tsp baking powder
- 1/4 tsp salt
- 1/3 cup milk
- 1 egg
- 2 tbsp unsalted butter, melted
- 1 tsp vanilla extract
- Vegetable oil for frying
- Toppings (optional): powdered sugar, cinnamon•sugar, chocolate glaze, sprinkles

Homemade donuts are a fun and delicious treat that kids will love. Encourage your young chef to experiment with different flavor combinations and toppings. Enjoy!

PROCEDURE:

1. In a large bowl, whisk together the flour, sugar, baking powder, and salt.

2. In a separate bowl, whisk together the milk, egg, melted butter, and vanilla.

3. Pour the wet ingredients into the dry ingredients and stir just until combined. Do not overmix.

4. On a lightly floured surface, roll the dough out to about 1/2•inch thickness.

5. Use a donut cutter or two different sized round cookie cutters to cut out the donut shapes.

6. In a large pot or Dutch oven, heat 2•3 inches of vegetable oil to 350°F.

7. Carefully add the donut shapes to the hot oil and fry for 1•2 minutes per side, until golden brown.

8. Remove the fried donuts from the oil using a slotted spoon and place them on a paper towel•lined plate to drain.

9. While the donuts are still warm, toss them in powdered sugar, cinnamon•sugar, or dip them in a chocolate glaze. Top with sprinkles if desired.

113. DECORATED SUGAR COOKIES

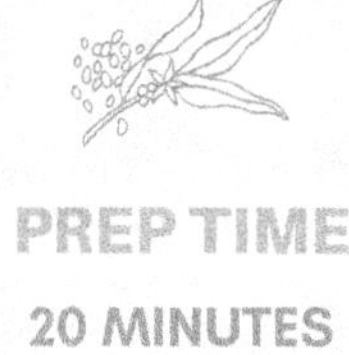

PREP TIME
20 MINUTES

COOK TIME
30 MINUTES

INGREDIENTS :

- 2 cups all•purpose flour
- 1/2 tsp baking powder
- 1/4 tsp salt
- 1 cup unsalted butter, softened
- 1 cup granulated sugar
- 1 egg
- 1 tsp vanilla extract

Icing:
- 2 cups powdered sugar
- 2•3 tbsp milk or water
- Food coloring (optional)

9. Make the icing: In a medium bowl, whisk together the powdered sugar and 2 tbsp of milk or water until smooth. Add more milk/water as needed to reach your desired consistency. Divide the icing into separate bowls and add food coloring, if desired. Use a spoon, knife, or piping bag to decorate the cooled cookies.

PROCEDURE :

1. In a medium bowl, whisk together the flour, baking powder, and salt. Set aside.

2. In a large bowl, beat the butter and sugar together until light and fluffy, about 2•3 minutes. Beat in the egg and vanilla.

3. Gradually add the dry ingredients to the wet ingredients, mixing until just combined. Do not overmix.

4. Divide the dough in half, shape each half into a disk, wrap in plastic wrap, and refrigerate for at least 1 hour (or up to 3 days).

5. Preheat the oven to 350°F (175°C). Line baking sheets with parchment paper.

6. Roll out the dough on a lightly floured surface to about 1/4•inch thickness. Use cookie cutters to cut out shapes.

7. Carefully transfer the cookies to the prepared baking sheets, spacing them about 1 inch apart.

8. Bake for 8•10 minutes, until the edges are just starting to lightly brown. Allow the cookies to cool on the baking sheets for 5 minutes before transferring to a wire rack to cool completely.

114. CUPCAKE CONES

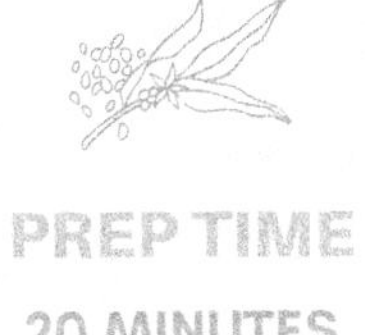

PREP TIME
20 MINUTES

COOK TIME
30 MINUTES

INGREDIENTS:

• 1 box of your favorite cake mix
(plus ingredients to make the cake)
• Cupcake liners or ice cream cones
• Frosting (store•bought or
homemade)
• Sprinkles, candies, or other
decorations (optional)

**This is a great recipe for young
chefs because:**

• They can help measure and mix
the cake batter

• They can fill the cupcake liners or
ice cream cones

• They can frost the cooled
cupcakes or cone cakes

• They can get creative with the
decoration

PROCEDURE:

1. Preheat your oven according to the cake mix
instructions.

2. Prepare the cake batter according to the
instructions on the box.

3. If using cupcake liners, place them in a muffin
tin. If using ice cream cones, stand them up in a
muffin tin or on a baking sheet.

4. Carefully fill the cupcake liners or ice cream
cones about 3/4 full with the cake batter.

5. Bake the cupcakes or cone cakes for the time
recommended on the cake mix box, usually 18•22
minutes.

6. Allow the cupcakes or cone cakes to cool
completely before frosting.

7. Once cooled, frost the cupcakes or cone cakes
with your desired frosting.

8. Decorate the frosted cupcakes or cone cakes
with sprinkles, candies, or other toppings, if
desired.

115. ICE CREAM SANDWICHES

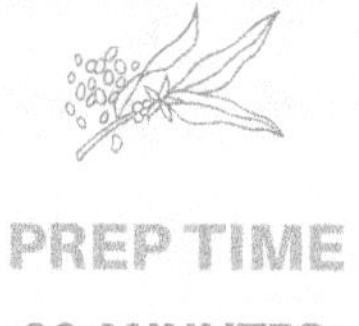 

PREP TIME
20 MINUTES

COOK TIME
30 MINUTES

INGREDIENTS:

• 1 box of your favorite cookie or brownie mix (plus ingredients to make the cookies/brownies)
• 1 quart of your favorite ice cream, softened

his is a great recipe for young chefs because:

• They can help measure and mix the cookie or brownie batter

• They can scoop the batter onto the baking sheet

• They can assemble the ice cream sandwiches by placing the ice cream between the cookies or brownies

• They can wrap the sandwiches and place them in the freezer

PROCEDURE:

1. Preheat your oven according to the cookie or brownie mix instructions.

2. Prepare the cookie or brownie batter according to the instructions on the box.

3. Scoop the batter onto a baking sheet, spacing the cookies or brownie squares about 2 inches apart.

4. Bake the cookies or brownies for the time recommended on the box, usually 8•12 minutes for cookies and 20•25 minutes for brownies.

5. Allow the cookies or brownies to cool completely on the baking sheet.

6. Once cooled, place a scoop of softened ice cream onto the flat side of one cookie or brownie square.

7. Top the ice cream with another cookie or brownie square, pressing down gently to create a sandwich.

8. Wrap each ice cream sandwich individually in plastic wrap or foil and place them in the freezer for at least 2 hours, or until firm.

Congratulations on reaching the end of ***"110+ Recipes Cookbook for Young Chefs: Simple Step-by-Step Instructions for Aspiring Cooks"!*** By exploring the recipes and techniques in this book, you've taken significant steps toward becoming a more confident and skilled chef. Your journey through these pages has been about more than just following recipes; it's been about discovering the joy and creativity of cooking.

Reflecting on Your Journey

Think back to when you first opened this cookbook. You may have felt a mix of excitement and nervousness, wondering what culinary adventures awaited you. As you've worked through the recipes, you've likely encountered new ingredients, tried different cooking methods, and perhaps even made a few mistakes along the way. Each experience, whether a triumph or a challenge, has contributed to your growth as a young chef.

Beyond the Recipes

While this cookbook has provided you with over 110 delicious recipes, the skills and knowledge you've gained extend far beyond these pages. You now have the confidence to experiment in the kitchen, the curiosity to try new foods, and the ability to prepare meals that bring joy to yourself and others.

Keep Cooking and Learning

Remember, cooking is a lifelong journey. There's always something new to learn, a new recipe to try, or a new technique to master. Don't be afraid to continue exploring and expanding your culinary horizons. Whether you're cooking for yourself, your family, or your friends, the skills you've developed will always serve you well.

A Note of Thanks

Thank you for choosing this cookbook as your guide. It's been an honor to accompany you on your culinary adventure. We hope that the recipes and tips in this book have inspired you and that you continue to find joy in cooking for many years to come.

Final Thoughts

As you close this book, take pride in all that you've accomplished. You are now equipped with the knowledge and skills to create delicious, homemade meals with confidence. So, keep experimenting, keep learning, and most importantly, keep cooking! Your culinary journey has just begun, and we can't wait to see where it takes you.

Happy cooking, young chef!